ARTHRITIS SURVIVAL

Other books by Robert S. Ivker, D.O.

Sinus Survival
The Self-Care Guide to Holistic Medicine
Thriving

ARTHRITIS SURVIVAL

THE HOLISTIC MEDICAL TREATMENT PROGRAM FOR OSTEOARTHRITIS

ROBERT S. IVKER, D.O.
and TODD NELSON, N.D.

Jeremy P. Tarcher/Putnam
a member of Penguin Putnam Inc.
NEW YORK

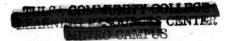

Most Tarcher/Putnam books are available at special quantity discounts for bulk purchase for sales promotions, premiums, fund-raising, and educational needs. Special books or book excerpts also can be created to fit specific needs. For details, write Putnam Special Markets, 375 Hudson Street, New York, NY 10014.

Jeremy P. Tarcher/Putnam
a member of
Penguin Putnam Inc.
375 Hudson Street
New York, NY 10014
www.penguinputnam.com

Library of Congress Cataloging-in-Publication Data

Ivker, Robert S.
   Arthritis survival : the holistic medical treatment program
for osteoarthritis / Robert S. Ivker and Todd Nelson.
      p.   cm.
   ISBN 1-58542-097-2
      1. Osteoarthritis—Alternative treatment.
   2. Holistic medicine.   I. Nelson, Todd.   II. Title.

   RC931.O67 I95   2001   00-053263
   616.7'22306—dc21

Printed in the United States of America

10   9   8   7   6   5   4   3   2   1

This book is printed on acid-free paper. ∞

To Thriving

ACKNOWLEDGMENTS

I am extremely grateful to my publisher, Joel Fotinos, for providing me with the opportunity to share holistic medicine with the millions of arthritis sufferers so desperately in need of hope. I'd also like to thank my literary agent, Gail Ross, for originally proposing the idea of writing a "survival guide series" (Arthritis, Asthma, Headache, and Backache) to follow the successful lead of *Sinus Survival*. In addition, I would like to acknowledge my co-authors of *The Self-Care Guide to Holistic Medicine,* Bob Anderson and Larry Trivieri, Jr. Many of their valuable contributions to that book have been incorporated into *Arthritis Survival*.

Most of all, I'd like to recognize my co-author, colleague, and friend, Todd Nelson, for his unwavering commitment and effort on this project. The expertise he's gained from the successful holistic treatment of arthritis patients during the past eighteen years of practice has been a critical ingredient in the formulation of the Arthritis Survival Program. The synergy of working so closely with a fellow healer and kindred spirit has made this both an educational and exhilarating project. Thank you, Todd.

CONTENTS

ARTHRITIS SURVIVAL

INTRODUCTION

"Only when we are sick of our sickness shall we cease to be sick."

LAO-TSU, from the *Tao Te Ching*

This book is based on the model of holistic medical treatment for chronic disease that I originally developed in the best-selling book *Sinus Survival*. Both of these books describe a holistic program of self-healing and optimal health that includes a comprehensive guide to therapeutic options for treating, preventing, and potentially curing the specific condition. The focus of this book is osteoarthritis or simply, arthritis.

Holistic medicine is defined as *the art and science of healing that addresses the whole person—body, mind, and spirit. Holistic physicians use both conventional and alternative therapies to prevent and treat disease, but—most importantly—to promote optimal health.* In the following chapters I will present information to help you treat, prevent, and heal your arthritis as well as experience optimal well-being. This will include:

- symptoms and diagnosis
- conventional medical treatment
- risk factors and causes
- holistic medical treatment and prevention, with recommendations for body, mind, and spirit (including *diet, nutritional*

supplements, herbs, and specific *physical, psychological,* and *bioenergetic therapies).*

The most basic principle in practicing holistic medicine is that *unconditional love is life's most powerful healer.* The primary objective of this book is, therefore, to teach you how to **love, nurture, and rejuvenate the chronically inflamed and painful joint surfaces,** which are probably causing you enough discomfort to significantly diminish the quality of your life. I'm assuming that's why you bought the book. But, in addition to reversing the symptoms of arthritis, it will be possible for you to experience a condition of **holistic health**—to feel better than you have in many years, while you relieve the pain and swelling in your joints.

Bear in mind as you begin to implement this holistic treatment program that *true healing is far greater than simply the absence of illness.* The most effective way to cure any chronic illness is to *heal your life,* not just repair your physical dysfunction, which in your case is probably painful and stiff joints, neck, or back. Therefore, I strongly advise that you use most of the tools and information provided in chapters 3, 4, 5, and 6—"Holistic Health: The Wellness Self-Test"; "Healing Your Body"; "Healing Your Mind"; and "Healing Your Spirit"—and not just simply rely on the Quick Fix in Chapter 1. What you learn in the latter chapters will assist you in strengthening your immune system and increasing your awareness of the physical, environmental, mental, emotional, spiritual, and social factors that may be contributing to your arthritis. The specific therapies provided in these chapters will then enable you to more permanently reverse the symptoms and prevent recurrences, rather than experience a temporary fix. *The holistic treatment of any chronic disease includes addressing and eliminating the multiple causes; adhering to a healthy diet; getting regular exercise; making affirmations, visualizations, emotional work, prayer, or meditation a part of your life; and creating intimate relationships.* As a result, you will become much more sensitive to what foods, thoughts, feelings, or people make you feel good, and those that make you feel more uncomfortable or even aggravate your arthritis. You can begin your training as a healer of your arthritis by first relieving your discomfort by following the recommendations in Chapter 1, "The Arthritis 'Quick-Fix'"; gaining a greater understanding of what arthritis is in Chapter 2; and taking the Wellness Self-Test in Chapter 3. Then you will be ready to start the Arthritis Survival Program in Chapter 4.

WORKING WITH YOUR PHYSICIAN

Although this book is intended as a self-care guide to healing arthritis and creating optimal wellness, I recognize that many people will read it while under the care of a physician. I recommend that you use the suggested therapies as a *complement* to the medical treatment you may already be receiving, and urge you to inform your doctor that you are doing so. Nothing in this book contradicts conventional medical treatment, and *proper drug use under the guidance of your physician can be practiced safely in conjunction with the holistic therapies I provide, unless specifically stated.* Holistic physicians recognize that drugs and surgery play an important role in treating disease, and I have included a section on the conventional medical treatment for arthritis. My therapeutic recommendations are based on the successful approaches that I, Todd Nelson, N.D. (the co-creator of the Arthritis Survival Program), and many of our holistic medical colleagues use to treat arthritis in our clinical practices. By following these recommendations, over time you will experience considerable improvement in your arthritic condition, with great potential for freeing yourself of this disabling condition and feeling healthier than you ever have before. The comprehensive focus on healing all of the life issues that may be contributing to your arthritis lies at the heart of the practice of holistic medicine and is the essence of the term *self-care.*

WORKING ON YOUR OWN

If you are not already under a physician's care, you might try starting with the holistic therapies on your own, unless otherwise indicated, and see how you feel after two months, before deciding to use conventional treatment or finding a holistic physician. And if you have been treated conventionally and conclude, after careful consideration and consultation with your physician, that the liabilities of the conventional treatment (such as toxic side effects of medication or surgical risks) outweigh their potential benefits, then commit solely to the holistic approach presented in the book, or take steps to find a holistic physician. One of the advantages of holistic medicine is that its combined use of complementary and conventional therapies often makes it possible to use lower dosages of medications to good effect, thereby minimizing harmful side effects.

HOLISTIC PHYSICIANS

If you are suffering from arthritis (or any other chronic disease) or trying to improve the quality of your life, you may want the support of a holistic physician. You can find one in your area by contacting the American Holistic Medical Association (AHMA) on their Web site *www.holisticmedicine.org* to obtain their *Physician Referral Directory*. This list includes both physician members (M.D.'s and D.O.'s) and associate members (holistic practitioners other than M.D.'s and D.O.'s). The best resource for a referral to a *board-certified* holistic physician is the American Board of Holistic Medicine (ABHM). On December 7, 2000, the ABHM administered the first certification examination in holistic medicine to nearly 300 physicians—M.D.'s and D.O.'s. The ABHM may be contacted at (425) 741-2996.

PROFESSIONAL COMPLEMENTARY THERAPIES

The discipline of holistic medicine includes the prudent use of both conventional Western medicine and professional care alternatives, such as *ayurveda, acupuncture, behavioral medicine, Chinese medicine, chiropractic, energy medicine, environmental medicine, homeopathy, naturopathic medicine, nutritional medicine,* and *osteopathic medicine.* Chapters 4, 5, and 6 include mention of each of these therapies, which have been scientifically verified as appropriate professional care treatments for arthritis. To learn more about these therapies, see the Resource Guide, which lists the primary organizations that oversee each of these therapies and provides a listing of practitioners nationwide. Each of them is also described in the Appendix of *The Self-Care Guide to Holistic Medicine.*

CHARTING YOUR PROGRESS

One way to monitor the progress of your holistic treatment program for arthritis is to evaluate your physical symptoms on a weekly basis. You can do so by using a chart similar to the Symptom Chart shown on pages 29–30. This is an example of a "musculoskeletal disease" symptom chart, and lists the most common symptoms you may experience if you suffer from arthritis, arthralgia, back or neck pain. If you experience symptoms not included on this list, then add them in the left-hand column and rank them from 1 (worst) to 10 (best = normal, i.e., no symptom) on a weekly basis. You can also uncover possible emotional factors that are contributing to your condition by similarly ranking your emotional stress level each week. You should be able to graphically correlate higher stress with worsening physical symptoms. The same is often true with dietary factors. Also keep track of the medications, herbs, nutritional supplements, and other remedies you are using at the bottom of the chart.

Note: The vitamins, herbs, and supplements recommended in chapter 4 are available in most health food stores and through Sinus Survival & Thriving Health Products. The suggested dosages are based upon those that I, Todd Nelson, N.D., and our holistic colleagues have used extensively in our clinical practices. These dosages may vary from the suggestions of your own personal holistic physician.

By using the Symptom Chart you can more easily evaluate your progress and better determine what works for you and what doesn't. (Remember, each of us is a unique individual, with specific needs and requirements for health.) As you practice using this chart you'll become quite adept at the early recognition of dietary, environmental, and emotional factors that aggravate your arthritis, and be able to quickly respond with an effective therapy. The better you become at listening attentively to your body, mind, and spirit, the more effectively you will be able to *prevent* recurrences of your condition. This art, science, and discipline is the basis for the practice of both holistic and preventive medicine. As you continue your training you will develop into a highly skilled self-healer. Although you may be starting out suffering with arthritis, remember that *the greater your enjoyment of this life-changing challenge, the better your results will be.*

This book will enlighten and educate you: You'll learn why you've felt so miserable for so long, and what you can do to improve that condition. But for the Arthritis Survival Program to make a profound difference in your life, you'll need to give yourself a gentle but firm push in the direction of optimal health—a condition of high energy and vitality, creativity, peace of mind, self-awareness, self-acceptance, passion, and intimacy. The critical ingredients for your success are a heightened *awareness* of your needs and desires (What do want your life to be like?); a *commitment* to providing them for yourself; the *time* required to incorporate new healthy habits into your life; and the *discipline* to stay on your course in spite of pain and disability.

These are the essential factors in learning to love and nurture yourself, and especially your joints. And it is also the primary objective of this holistic medical treatment program.

If you are willing to make the commitment, this program will enable you to *heal yourself of arthritis.* Although you may still have an occasional arthritis flare-up, you will no longer experience chronic pain or significant disability. More importantly, you will understand why the arthritis attack occurs, have the tools to treat it quickly, and avoid being in pain for a prolonged period of time. But the most significant aspect of your healing process is that you will almost always learn or re-learn a valuable lesson through your discomfort that helps to *prevent* subsequent attacks.

Although optimal health requires a commitment to a lifelong healing *process,* we live in an age of the quick fix. We've grown up believing that there's a fast and effortless solution to all of life's hardships. And if there is not such a miracle available today, it won't be long before science and technology provide it. But to heal your deteriorating joints, while creating a balance of optimal well-being throughout every dimension of your life, requires a commitment to the Arthritis Survival Program comparable to one you'd make if you'd just started a new job. *Healing yourself is the most important work you'll ever do, and the greatest gift you'll ever receive.*

After two months of making a commitment to this program, you will probably be "surviving" quite well, with a significant improvement in your symptoms. If you can maintain and strengthen that commitment to yourself, within six months you will be healthier than you've been in years, and within one year you'll be experiencing a state of well-being you've never known before. The most important advice I can give you is to take your time, be gentle and accepting of yourself, and know that there are no mistakes—only lessons. Study diligently, listen attentively, be willing to take risks, and have fun while you're at it. It's definitely a challenge, but the rewards are unimaginable!

Rob Ivker
November 2000

Chapter 1

THE ARTHRITIS "QUICK FIX"

Since I've described the Arthritis Survival Program in the Introduction as a *healing process* and not a quick fix, you may be wondering about the title of this chapter. Yet, when attempting to make a significant change in our lives, most of us need a simple, safe, and effective way to get started, along with the prospect for seeing some positive results relatively soon. In our modern, high-tech society we've been conditioned to believe there's a quick-fix solution to almost all of our needs and desires. If you suffer from arthritis, however, you've probably already realized that there isn't such a thing for your condition or any other chronic ailment. The following recommendations are the most frequent suggestions Dr. Nelson and I offer our patients for relief of symptoms in the shortest period of time. It is based on extensive scientific research and consistent clinical outcomes.

The Quick Fix is an abbreviated version of the physical health component of the Arthritis Survival Program, described in much more depth in Chapter 4. If you'd like more information on obtaining specific products, please refer to the Product Index on page 207. Since you will probably not choose to do everything on this list, we would strongly advise you to refer to Chapter 4 in selecting the therapeutic options that feel right for you in beginning the Arthritis Survival Program. You can begin any or all aspects of the Quick Fix recommendations immediately at your discretion. As always, we advise you to make your health professionals aware of your choices.

VITAMINS, MINERALS, AND SUPPLEMENTS

- **glucosamine sulfate**—1,000mg 3x/day for 12 weeks, followed by a maintenance dosage of 500mg 3x/day. This supplement is considered safe, but it can occasionally produce heartburn and diarrhea. It usually takes 4 to 8 weeks to get significant benefit from glucosamine.
- **chondroitin sulfate**—400mg 3x/day.
- **SAMe (S-adenosylmethionine)**—400mg 3x/day for 21 days, then reduce to 200mg 2x/day.
- **MSM (methylsulfonylmethane)**—300 to 500mg 2x/day.
- **collagen**—dosage varies with brand.
- **Essential fatty acids (EFAs)**—EPA (eicosapentaenoic acid) in a dosage of up to 600mg 4x/day for 12 weeks, then reduce to 3x/day; DHA (docosahexaenoic acid), up to 400mg 4x/day for 2 months, then reduce to 3x/day; and flaxseed oil, 1 tablespoon 2x/day with meals or 3 capsules 3x/day with meals.
- **vitamin C**—1,000 to 6,000mg/day, in an ascorbate form or Ester-C.
- **vitamin A**—10,000 to 25,000 IU/day.
- **vitamin E**—400 to 1,200 IU/day as natural d-alpha-tocopherol.
- **vitamin B complex**—50 to 100mg/day.
- **grape-seed extract (proanthocyanidin)**—100 to 300mg/day.
- **zinc arginate or glycinate**—50mg/day.
- **selenium**—200mcg/day.
- **copper aspirinate**—2mg/day.
- **calcium (MCHA type)**—1,000mg/day.
- **magnesium glycinate**—500mg/day.
- **manganese**—30mg/day.
- **niacinamide (vitamin B$_3$)**—250 to 500mg 3x/day.
- **methionine**—200mg 3x/day.

- **L-glutamine**—5 grams 2x/day in powder form.
- **NAC (N-acetylcysteine)**—200 to 800mg/day.
- **enzymes (chymotrypsin, pancreatin, and bromelain)**—taken with each meal.
- **bioflavanoids (including quercetin)**—500mg 3x/day.
- **probiotics (consisting of *Lactobacillus acidophilus* and *Bifidobacterium*)**—½ teaspoon or 2 capsules 3x/day, preferably on an empty stomach.

DIET

Eliminate:

- **nightshade plants**—potatoes, peppers, eggplant, tomatoes, and tobacco
- **dairy products**
- **wheat**
- **all animal products other than fish and DHA-enhanced eggs**
- **alcohol**
- **coffee and caffeine**
- **sugar, soda pop, sweeteners of any kind (including artificial)**
- **saturated fat, hydrogenated fat (margarine), and fried foods**
- **processed and refined foods**
- **excess salt**
- **white flour products**
- **spinach**
- **cranberries**
- **plums**
- **white and other distilled vinegars, except raw apple-cider vinegar, which can be helpful**
- **citrus fruits, except lemon.**

Include:

- **hypo-allergenic, nutrient-dense diet emphasizing a high volume of raw fruits and vegetables and minimal**

amounts of flesh of land animals, i.e., red meat and poultry

- **green leafy and high water content vegetables**—3 to 6 cups daily (See Chapter 4 for complete list.)
- **raw vegetable juices**—diluted to 30 percent with pure water
- **water**—pure (filtered or bottled), 6 to 8 glasses per day (Drink between meals.)
- **carrots**
- **avocado**
- **seaweeds**
- **spirulina**
- **barley and wheat grass products**
- **sprouts**
- **pecans**
- **soy products**
- **whole grains**—such as brown rice, millet, oats, quinoa, amaranth, and barley.
- **seeds**—sesame, flax, and pumpkin
- **cold-water fish**—such as salmon, sardines, herring, halibut, sole, cod, and tuna
- **eggs**—from organically fed free-range chickens whose yolks are DHA-enhanced as a result of the chickens eating brown algae.

Weight reduction, through diet and exercise, is also strongly recommended in treating arthritis.

HERBS

- **boswellia**—500mg standardized to 70 percent boswellic acids, 3 to 5x/day between meals.
- **curcumin** *(Curcurma longa)*—an extract of the common spice **turmeric,** 250 to 400mg containing 95 percent curcuminoids 3x/day between meals and combined with 1,000mg of bromelain.
- **devil's claw** *(Harpagphytum procumbens)*—1 to 2 grams, 3x/day.

- **cayenne (capsaicin)**—available as an OTC cream containing the active ingredient capsaicin, for analgesia: Apply directly to affected joints 3 or 4x/day for at least a week; also available as a capsule, 500mg 3x/day.
- **ginger** *(Zingiber officinale)*—0.5 to 1mg of powdered ginger daily or as a tea (one grated teaspoon of fresh ginger in a cup of hot water, 2x/day). More simply, you may take a standardized extract (5% or more gingerol) of ginger combined with 500 to 1,000mg of mixed bioflavanoids or include it in your diet.
- **white willow bark**—for acute pain, 4:1 standardized extract, 200 to 400mg 3x/day between meals.
- **licorice root** *(Glycyrrhiza glabra)*—⅛ to ¼ of a teaspoon of a 5:1 solid extract up to 3x/day. Licorice used long-term can elevate blood pressure and increase potassium loss.
- **castor oil hot packs**—apply to affected joint.

EXERCISE

Good choices for *low-impact exercise* are:

- **walking**
- **swimming**
- **cycling**—at low pedal resistance, over level surfaces at first
- **rowing**
- **water walking**
- **aqua aerobics**
- **ballroom or other low-impact dancing.**
- **Pilates**—an exercise system based on yoga, the use of specialized equipment, and a mind/body focus.

Chapter 2

WHAT IS ARTHRITIS? WHAT CAUSES IT? HOW DOES CONVENTIONAL MEDICINE TREAT IT?

According to the National Center for Health Statistics, arthritis afflicts approximately 35 million Americans or about 13 percent of the population, ranking it as our second most common chronic disease, behind sinusitis. By 2020 it is projected to afflict about 18 percent of the populace. It is characterized by painful, stiff, or swollen joints. *Osteoarthritis,* also known as *degenerative arthritis* or *degenerative joint disease,* is the most common type of joint disease (about 21 million sufferers) and is the subject of this book. It rarely begins before the age of 40 (when it does, it's much more common in men), but an estimated 50 to 80 percent of people over the age of 65 have some degree of arthritis. Throughout the book, whenever I use the word *arthritis,* I am referring to osteoarthritis. It differs significantly from *rheumatoid arthritis* (about 7 million sufferers), which is caused primarily by inflammation, leads to severe joint deformity, and affects tissues in the body other than the joints.

ANATOMY AND PHYSIOLOGY

Arthritis usually affects a synovial joint—one that is encased in a tough fibrous capsule lined with a membrane that secretes a thick, clear synovial fluid. This type of joint connects one bone to another and, with the fluid lubricating the cartilaginous surfaces, allows for smooth motion. The cartilage, covering the ends of the bones, is made of a smooth, soft, cushionlike material that acts as a shock absorber and reduces friction by preventing the bones from rubbing against one another. *Arthritis is a progressive degeneration of the cartilage combined with the body's inability to regenerate the cartilage at the same pace.* In an arthritic joint there may either be insufficient synovial fluid, causing stiffness, or an excess, causing swelling. If the cartilage has broken down enough to allow the bones to rub against one another, there is significant pain. The body often attempts to repair the joint damage by producing bony outgrowths at the margins of the affected joints. These spurs can also cause pain and stiffness.

Since osteoarthritis is a disease of cartilage, let's take a closer look at this white, shiny, slippery, firm substance that functions as the body's primary shock absorber. Extremely strong and

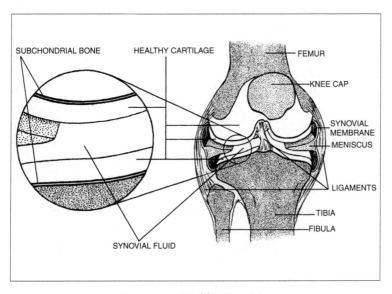

FIGURE 1.   *Healthy Knee Joint*

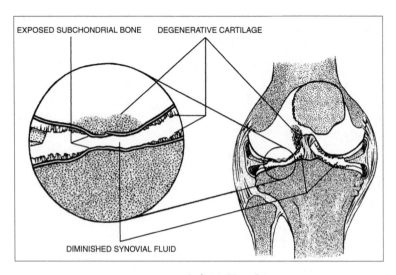

EXPOSED SUBCHONDRIAL BONE   DEGENERATIVE CARTILAGE

DIMINISHED SYNOVIAL FLUID

FIGURE 2.   *Arthritic Knee Joint*

flexible, cartilage is a specialized type of connective tissue that is found on the ends of bones and is eight times more slippery than ice. It is composed of 80 to 85 percent water; the rest consists of collagen, proteoglycans, and chondrocytes, which are described below. Although cartilage is a living substance that requires nourishment, it is one of the few tissues in the body that does *not* have its own blood supply. Therefore, it is dependent upon the synovial fluid that surrounds the joint to obtain nutrients.

Collagen, sometimes called the threads of cartilage, is made up of densely woven strands of amino acids built into chains of proteins; it provides shape and resiliency to cartilage. Called collagen type II, it is found only in cartilage.

Proteoglycans are large water-loving molecules that hold the threads of collagen together and help to nurture cartilage. When strung together, the proteoglycans together with collagen provides shape, size, and resiliency, along with the functions of cartilage as a gliding surface and shock absorber for the joints.

Chondrocytes are cells that act as the production center for cartilage, manufacturing both collagen and proteoglycans. They also produce enzymes that digest weakened collagen and proteoglycans. Since their primary function is to produce new and destroy old cartilage, the health of the chondrocytes is essential to maintaining healthy cartilage. Any factor that diminishes optimal function of the chondrocytes can contribute to causing degeneration of the cartilage and arthritis.

SYMPTOMS AND DIAGNOSIS

There are no definitive laboratory tests for arthritis. The diagnosis is usually made from a physical examination, an X ray, fluid withdrawn from a joint, and especially from the *medical history.* The primary symptoms of arthritis are:

- intermittent pain with motion of affected joints
- stiffness and limitation of movement, with audible cracking in the joints
- swelling and deformity of the joint
- pattern of gradual onset.

Arthritis pain tends to fluctuate with weather patterns, responding to both temperature and barometric changes. The degenerative changes of osteoarthritis can often be seen in the spine on X rays, but the majority of people with these changes do not have back pain.

Although *primary osteoarthritis,* the more common type, can occur in any joint in the body, it usually affects the fingers (particularly the two joints closest to the fingertips), the knees, hips, neck, and lower spine. The cause of primary osteoarthritis, usually described as "inflammation of the joints," is not known. While inflammation is often present to some extent, it does not appear to be the primary cause of the joint damage. It is also assumed by most physicians and patients suffering with arthritis that it is caused by progressive wear and tear on the joints, resulting in the gradual destruction of cartilage. As the joint disease gradually progresses, the cartilage cracks and flakes off, leading to subsequent pain, stiffness, and sometimes deformity whenever the underlying and now exposed bones rub together. However, although cartilage damage is one of the hallmarks of osteoarthritis, *heavy use of the joints does **not** necessarily cause problems.* In fact, many former long-distance runners have perfectly normal hips and knees, while their more sedentary friends may be suffering with degenerative joint disease.

Secondary osteoarthritis can occur after an injury to a joint, from disease, or as a result of chronic trauma, e.g., obesity, poor posture, or occupational overuse. With every chronic disease, it appears that *there is a combination of multiple factors that increase the risk of that condition occurring.* The same is true for both primary and secondary osteoarthritis.

RISK FACTORS AND CAUSES OF OSTEOARTHRITIS

Factors that increase the chances of developing osteoarthritis are:

- **heredity**
- **severe or recurrent joint injury from heavy physical activity**
- **skeletal postural defects and congenital joint instability**
- **obesity**—excessive body weight and high body mass index are significant predictors of osteoarthritis of the knee. In men, the risk for arthritis of the knee is 50 to 350 percent greater for those who are the heaviest compared to those of normal weight. This principle probably relates to other weight-bearing joints as well.
- **exercise**—there is some evidence that only the most violent joint-pounding activities (long-distance running, basketball, etc.) performed over many years will predispose to the development of arthritis.

- **cold climate and barometric pressure changes**
- **food allergy**—especially nightshades (potatoes, tomatoes, peppers, and eggplants), wheat, and dairy
- **a diet high in animal products**
- **nutrient deficiency**—lack of vitamin C, calcium, magnesium, manganese, protein, D-glucuronic acid, essential fatty acids
- **low-grade infections (e.g., dental infections) and autoimmune disease**
- **dehydration**
- **excessive acid in the body**—causing increased amounts of calcium, minerals, and acid toxins to be deposited in the joint, resulting in inflammation and pain
- **yeast overgrowth or candidiasis**
- **other systemic disorders often associated with arthritis**—including nutritional deficiencies, digestive disorders such as leaky gut syndrome, constipation, fatigue, emotional stress, and endocrine disorders

The specific mental and emotional issues often found in people with arthritis are: sensitivity to criticism, low self-esteem and self-confidence, feeling unloved, lack of trust, resentment, and fear and intimidation.

Each of these potential causes (other than heredity) is addressed in the Arthritis Survival Program, the holistic medical treatment for arthritis described in chapters 4, 5, and 6.

CONVENTIONAL MEDICAL TREATMENT OF OSTEOARTHRITIS

The following are conventional recommendations for the treatment of osteoarthritis:

- **Reduction of stresses** on joints is usually advised, using a splint, a brace, a neck collar, crutches, or a cane. In addition, reducing or eliminating activities that expose the joint to repetitive, high-impact forces is also recommended. This is especially helpful for knees and hips, as is weight loss. Every pound of body weight lost reduces the force across the knee by five to ten pounds.
- **Physical therapy** is often prescribed, including exercise (swimming, water aerobics, walking, bicycling, and cross-country skiing, in addition to strengthening and stretching); hot and cold packs; diathermy; and paraffin baths.
- **Drugs** can minimize pain and inflammation if present. Treatment usually begins with acetaminophen (Tylenol) and progresses to nonsteroidal anti-inflammatory drugs (NSAIDs), which may either be prescription or over-the-counter. The most commonly recommended NSAIDs are ibuprofen (Advil, Nuprin), naproxen (Aleve, Naprosyn), nabumetone (Relafen), piroxicam (Feldene), and etodolac (Lodine). Aspirin is not recommended for osteoarthritis because the high doses needed to reduce pain may damage the stomach lining. The NSAIDs do not stop joint deterioration: In some instances they may even *accelerate* it by reducing a critical ingredient (glycosaminoglycans) in cartilage. Long-term use can also lead to a significant incidence of kidney and liver damage, capillary fragility, as well as stomach ulceration (and perforation) and small-bowel irritation. This is the leading cause of hospitalization due to ulcers of the stomach and duodenum, and leading cause of death resulting from complications of bleeding ulcer.

  The most recent arthritis drugs are the COX–2 selective inhibitors, celecoxib (Celebrex), and rofecoxib (Vioxx). These are also NSAIDs, and although no more effective in relieving pain than the drugs mentioned above, they seem to be less harmful to the gastrointestinal tract. They work by selectively blocking the COX–2 enzyme, which is believed responsible for the pain and inflammation of arthritis. Unlike traditional NSAIDs, however, they only minimally inhibit the COX–1 enzyme, which is instrumental in maintaining normal gastrointestinal and platelet function. The most likely candidates for COX–2 inhibitors are primarily patients who are at risk for NSAID-induced ulcers such as those with a history of bleeding ulcers.

The COX-2 drugs are considerably more expensive than the other NSAIDs.

Corticosteroids such as prednisone are used as a second-step drug to suppress the inflammation of arthritis. Long-term use tends to suppress immunity and diminishes production of the patient's own cortisone from the adrenal gland, accelerating degenerative changes such as osteoporosis.

• **Surgery,** which may be used as a late-stage intervention, may include reconstruction or replacement of hips (250,000 performed annually), knees (137,000 per year), knuckles, and other joints.

Hip replacement is an elective procedure that usually lasts between fifteen and twenty years. In spite of loss of mobility and the arthritic pain, people will often postpone this surgery until the pain begins to affect sleep. Best results occur with patients who are in good shape before surgery. This means weight loss and muscle-strengthening exercises. Water aerobics is often recommended prior to hip replacement. There are a wide variety of hip prostheses, depending upon the patient's age, activity level, and bone quality. Possible complications following surgery are blood clots (more common following hip and knee replacement than most other major surgeries), infection, and dislocation of the new hip. Several months of rehabilitation following surgery are the norm, and full recovery may take up to a year. About 95 percent of the patients who undergo the operation report significant pain relief and increased mobility. Most patients can expect to get back to even their more vigorous activities. The more fit you are prior to surgery, the more active you can be afterward.

Knee replacement is a painful operation requiring months of rigorous physical therapy following surgery. The surgery is usually recommended for people over 55 with a low to moderate activity level and whose pain seriously hampers day-to-day activity. Younger people are discouraged from having the surgery, since their higher level of overall activity would put excessive wear on an artificial knee, shortening its life span. Although knee replacement surgery is generally successful in relieving pain, in most cases it also significantly reduces mobility.

If only a small area of cartilage is damaged, as in some athletic injuries, and the person is highly active, the use of synthetic synovial fluid (called a viscosupplement) such as Synvisc may be considered. This material is injected into the joint space to provide temporary cushioning and pain relief.

- **Genetically engineered cartilage replacement** is a relatively new surgical procedure that appears to be quite promising. At the time of this writing, it has for the most part only been performed on arthritic knees, although physicians have just begun to experiment with elbows and shoulders. The procedure begins with the remaining healthy cartilage in a patient's knee being removed arthroscopically and sent to a genetic engineering laboratory in Boston. This specialized lab has developed the technique of regenerating cartilage. After growing in the laboratory for three months, the cartilage is then implanted in the patient's knee, and five months more are required for complete healing. Younger patients are preferred for this procedure since they are generally more active and the outcome is often a full range of mobility. It costs $25,000 and early results have been impressive. Olympic ski champion Picabo Street was able to resume ski racing following this cartilage replacement procedure.

Chapter 3

HOLISTIC HEALTH: THE WELLNESS SELF-TEST

"The only thing I know that truly heals people is unconditional love."

ELISABETH KÜBLER-ROSS, M.D.

Are you healthy? Your answer is probably "No, I have arthritis." But suppose you didn't, and let's also assume you have no other symptoms of disease, chronic ailment, or nagging condition that never quite goes away. If this were true, then you'd most likely respond, "Yes, I am healthy," since the conditioning that the majority of us have grown up with has taught us to define health as the absence of illness.

Yet, the words *health, heal,* and *holy* are all derived from the same Old English word, *hælan,* which means "to make whole." Viewed from this perspective, two questions that more directly and accurately address the issue of health are "Do you love your life?" and "Are you happy to be alive?"

Health is far more than simply a matter of not feeling ill: *It is the daily experience of wholeness and balance—a state of being fully alive in body, mind, and spirit.* Such a condition could also be called optimal, or *holistic,* health. I call it *thriving.* Helping you to achieve this state of total well-being is the primary objective of this book. *As a by-product of that healing process, the pain in your joints will subside and your arthritis will either improve significantly or be cured.* As you might imagine, this state of high-functioning well-being goes far beyond the conventional approach as outlined in Chapter 2, which focuses almost exclusively on symptom relief.

HALLMARKS OF OPTIMAL HEALTH

Optimal health results from harmony and balance in the physical, environmental, mental, emotional, spiritual, and social aspects of your life. When this harmonious balance is present, you can experience the *unlimited and unimpeded free flow of life force energy throughout your body, mind, and spirit.* Around the world, this energy is known by many names. The Chinese call it *qi* ("chee"), the Japanese refer to it as *ki,* in India it is known as *pranna,* and in Hebrew it is *chai.* But in the Western world, the phrase that comes closest to capturing the feeling generated by this energy is *unconditional love,* regarded by holistic physicians as *our most powerful healer.*

Although each of us has the capacity to nurture and to heal ourselves, most of us have yet to tap into this wellspring of loving life energy. Yet, there is no one who can better administer this life-enhancing elixir to you than you yourself.

By committing to caring for yourself in the manner recommended in the following chapters, you will in essence be learning how to better *give and receive love*—to yourself and others. As a result, you will be enhancing the flow of life force energy throughout every aspect of your life. This holistic healing process will also provide you with the opportunity to safely and effectively treat your arthritis and any other physical, mental, and spiritual conditions that may be impeding the flow of healing energy in your life.

Living a holistically healthy lifestyle can facilitate the realization of your ideal life vision in accordance with both your personal and professional goals. But since the majority of us are only aware of health as a condition of not being sick, a mental image of what living holistically means is needed in order to achieve it. Briefly, let's examine this state of optimal well-being to give you a glimpse of what it looks and feels like.

A list of the six components of health follows, the first italicized item in each category encompassing the essence of that component. For example, physical health can be simply described as a condition of *high energy and vitality,* while mental health is a state of *peace of mind and contentment.* The italicized items can also serve as a health gauge you can use to measure your progress in each area.

PHYSICAL HEALTH

High energy and vitality

- Freedom from, or high adaptability to, pain, dysfunction, and disability
- A strong immune system
- A body that feels light, balanced, strong, flexible, and has good aerobic capacity
- Ability to meet physical challenges and perform exceptionally
- Full capacity of all five senses and a healthy libido.

ENVIRONMENTAL HEALTH

Harmony with your environment (neither harming nor being harmed)

- Awareness of your connectedness with nature
- Feeling grounded—comfort and security within your surroundings
- Respect and appreciation for your home, the Earth and all of her inhabitants
- Contact with the earth; breathing healthy air; drinking pure water; eating uncontaminated food; exposure to the sun, fire, or candlelight; immersion in warm water (all on a daily basis).

MENTAL HEALTH

Peace of mind and contentment

- A job that you love doing
- Optimism

- A sense of humor
- Financial well-being
- Living your life vision
- The ability to express your creativity and talents
- The capacity to make healthy decisions.

EMOTIONAL HEALTH

Self-acceptance and high self-esteem

- Capacity to identify, express, experience, and accept all of your feelings, both painful and joyful
- Awareness of the intimate connection between your physical and emotional bodies
- The ability to confront your greatest fears
- The fulfillment of your capacity to play
- Peak experiences on a regular basis.

SPIRITUAL HEALTH

Experience of unconditional love/absence of fear

- Soul awareness and a personal relationship with God or Spirit
- Trust in your intuition and an openness to change
- Gratitude
- Creating a sacred space on a regular basis through prayer, meditation, walking in nature, observing a Sabbath day, or other rituals
- Sense of purpose
- Being present in every moment.

SOCIAL HEALTH

Intimacy with a spouse, partner, relative, or close friend

- Effective communication
- Forgiveness
- Sense of belonging to a support group or community
- Touch and/or physical intimacy on a daily basis
- Selflessness and altruism.

THE WELLNESS SELF-TEST

Now that you understand the six categories that constitute optimal health, it's time to measure how close you are to *thriving* in each area. The following questionnaire is designed to provide you with a much clearer idea of the status of your health in all six areas. You can use the results of the test to guide you through the rest of the book and it can become a blueprint for restructuring your life. You can also measure your progress by retaking the test every two or three months.

Answer the questions in each section below and total your score. Each response will be a number from 0 to 5. Please refer to the frequency described within the parentheses (e.g., "2 to 3x/wk") when answering questions about an *activity,* e.g., "Do you maintain a healthy diet?" However, when the question refers to an *attitude* or an *emotion* (most of the Mind and Spirit questions, e.g., "Do you have a sense of humor?"), the response is more subjective and less exact, and you should refer to the terms describing the frequency, such as *often* or *daily* but not to the numbered frequencies in parentheses:

0 = Never or almost never (once a year or less)
1 = Seldom (2 to 12x/year)
2 = Occasionally (2 to 4x/month)
3 = Often (2 to 3x/week)
4 = Regularly (4 to 6x/week)
5 = Daily (every day).

BODY: PHYSICAL AND ENVIRONMENTAL HEALTH

_____ 1. Do you maintain a healthy diet (low fat, low sugar, fresh fruits, grains and vegetables)?

_____ 2. Is your water intake adequate (at least ½ oz/lb of body weight; 160 lbs = 80 oz)?

_____ 3. Are you within 20 percent of your ideal body weight?

_____ 4. Do you feel physically attractive?

_____ 5. Do you fall asleep easily and sleep soundly?

_____ 6. Do you awaken in the morning feeling well rested?

_____ 7. Do you have more than enough energy to meet your daily responsibilities?

_____ 8. Are your five senses acute?

_____ 9. Do you take time to experience sensual pleasure?

_____10. Do you schedule regular massage or deep-tissue body work?

_____11. Does your sexual relationship feel gratifying?

_____12. Do you engage in regular physical workouts (lasting at least 20 minutes)?

_____13. Do you have good endurance or aerobic capacity?

_____14. Do you breathe abdominally for at least a few minutes?

_____15. Do you maintain physically challenging goals?

_____16. Are you physically strong?

_____17. Do you do some stretching exercises?

_____18. Are you free of chronic aches, pains, ailments, and diseases?

_____19. Do you have regular effortless bowel movements?

_____20. Do you understand the causes of your chronic physical problems?

_____21. Are you free of any drug (including caffeine and nicotine) or alcohol dependency?

_____22. Do you live and work in a healthy environment with respect to clean air, water, and indoor pollution?

_____23. Do you feel energized or empowered by nature?

_____24. Do you feel a strong connection with and appreciation for your body, your home, and your environment?

_____25. Do you have an awareness of life-energy or *qi* (chee)?

_____ TOTAL BODY SCORE

MIND: MENTAL AND EMOTIONAL HEALTH

_____ 1. Do you have specific goals in your personal and professional life?

_____ 2. Do you have the ability to concentrate for extended periods of time?

_____ 3. Do you use visualization or mental imagery to help you attain your goals or enhance your performance?

_____ 4. Do you believe it is possible to change?

_____ 5. Can you meet your financial needs and desires?

_____ 6. Is your outlook basically optimistic?

_____ 7. Do you give yourself more supportive messages than critical messages?

_____ 8. Does your job utilize all of your greatest talents?

_____ 9. Is your job enjoyable and fulfilling?

_____10. Are you willing to take risks or make mistakes in order to succeed?

_____11. Are you able to adjust beliefs and attitudes as a result of learning from painful experiences?

_____12. Do you have a sense of humor?

_____13. Do you maintain peace of mind and tranquillity?

_____14. Are you free from a strong need for control or the need to be right?

_____15. Are you able to fully experience (feel) your painful feelings, such as fear, anger, sadness, and hopelessness?

_____16. Are you aware of and able to safely express fear?

_____17. Are you aware of and able to safely express anger?

_____18. Are you aware of and able to safely express sadness (or cry)?

_____19. Are you accepting of all your feelings?

_____20. Do you engage in meditation, contemplation, or psychotherapy to better understand your feelings?

_____21. Is your sleep free from disturbing dreams?

_____22. Do you explore the symbolism and emotional content of your dreams?

_____23. Do you take the time to relax, or make time for activities that constitute the abandon or absorption of play?

_____24. Do you experience feelings of exhilaration?

_____25. Do you enjoy high self-esteem?

_____ TOTAL MIND SCORE

SPIRIT: SPIRITUAL AND SOCIAL HEALTH

_____ 1. Do you actively commit time to your spiritual life?

_____ 2. Do you take time for prayer, meditation, or reflection?

_____ 3. Do you listen and act upon your intuition?

_____ 4. Are creative activities a part of your work or leisure time?

_____ 5. Do you take risks?

_____ 6. Do you have faith in a God, spirit guides, or angels?

_____ 7. Are you free from anger toward God?

_____ 8. Are you grateful for the blessings in your life?

_____ 9. Do you take walks, garden, or have contact with Nature?

_____10. Are you able to let go of your attachment to specific outcomes and embrace uncertainty?

_____11. Do you observe a day of rest completely free of work, dedicated to nurturing yourself and your family?

_____12. Can you let go of self-interest in deciding the best course of action for a given situation?

_____13. Do you feel a sense of purpose?

_____14. Do you make time to connect with young children, either your own or someone else's?

_____15. Are playfulness and humor important to you in your daily life?

_____16. Do you have the ability to forgive yourself and others?

_____17. Have you demonstrated the willingness to commit to a marriage or comparable long-term relationship?

_____18. Do you experience intimacy, besides sex, in your committed relationships?

_____19. Do you confide in or speak openly with one or more close friends?

_____20. Do you or did you feel close to your parents?

_____21. If you have experienced the loss of a loved one, have you fully grieved that loss?

_____22. Has your experience of pain enabled you to grow spiritually?

_____23. Do you go out of your way or give your time to help others?

_____24. Do you feel a sense of belonging to a group or community?

_____25. Do you experience unconditional love?

_____ TOTAL SPIRIT SCORE

_____ TOTAL BODY, MIND, SPIRIT SCORE

HEALTH SCALE

325–375	Optimal health = THRIVING
275–324	Excellent health
225–274	Good health
175–224	Fair health
125–174	Below-average health
75–124	Poor health
Less than 75	Extremely unhealthy = SURVIVING

Once you complete this questionnaire, pay attention to which categories you need to make the most improvements in, and remember that *there are multiple factors that have combined to cause your arthritis.* Then start to implement the tools and suggestions that are outlined in chapters 4, 5, and 6. Chapter 4 gives you a blueprint for improving your physical and environmental health while also specifically addressing arthritis; Chapter 5 outlines similar approaches for mental and emotional health and looks at the most common emotional factors contributing to arthritis; while Chapter 6 will help you enhance your spiritual and social health. Begin where you are most comfortable and take your time. You are committing to a life-changing process, one that requires patience and discipline, so proceed at your own pace. Remember, too, that everyone is unique and no two of us will follow the exact same healing path. While the science of holistic medicine provides a universal foundation and structure, its *art* lies in the writing of your own personal prescription for optimal health, so feel free to adapt the techniques in the pages ahead to tailor-make the holistic self-care program that is most ideally suited for you. Your heart will be your primary guide on this odyssey of realizing your full potential as a human being.

Chapter 4

HEALING YOUR BODY
The Physical and Environmental Health Components of the Arthritis Survival Program

I f you would rather not learn to live with your arthritis, along with its diminished quality of life, then I would like to take you on a healing journey into an exciting new, yet ancient, frontier of medicine. For the past thirteen years, I have been practicing **holistic medicine** while treating arthritis, sinusitis, backache, headache, and a variety of other so-called chronic or "incurable" conditions. The Arthritis Survival Program has its foundation in the holistic practice of treating, preventing, and potentially curing any chronic condition, as well as creating a state of optimal well-being. Although the bulk of the holistic approach is similar for any chronic condition or disease, this and the following chapters include specific dietary, nutritional supplement, herbal recommendations, professional care therapies, as well as emotional factors that relate directly to treating the *causes and symptoms* of arthritis. *Commitment* to this approach has resulted in a significant improvement of the symptoms of arthritis, in addition to a far greater experience of well-being in many people. This success stems primarily from the basic *health* orientation of the holistic approach. Rather than focusing on the disease and just treating its symptoms—they are certainly not ignored, just perceived differently—holistic medicine addresses *causes* while restoring balance and harmony to the *whole person*. It goes far beyond the "quick fix" outlined in Chapter 1 or the repair of a "broken part," to an understanding of *what can be learned from your physical pain and how to use that knowledge to change your life and be free of arthritis.*

In my own case, I was led to the practice of holistic medicine and a condition of optimal health by my painful sinuses. My guide on this healing path was, and still is, Hippocrates, who recognized 2,500 years ago the most direct and effective method for training to become a healer: "Physician, heal thyself." In the remainder of this book, I'd like to guide you on a similar path leading, not only to the healing of your degenerative joint disease and any other dis-ease, but to a state of holistic health. By taking the Wellness Self-Test in Chapter 3, you have measured your present state of well-being. I'd recommend repeating this test every two to three months to gauge your physical, mental, and spiritual health progress and in your training as a healer of yourself.

In the process of healing your body along with your painful joints, the ultimate objective is the following state of physical and environmental well-being:

PHYSICAL HEALTH

High energy and vitality

- Freedom from, or high adaptability to, pain, dysfunction, and disability
- A strong immune system
- A body that feels light, balanced, strong, and flexible, and has good aerobic capacity
- Ability to meet physical challenges and perform exceptionally
- Full capacity of all five senses and a healthy libido.

Environmental Health

Harmony with your environment—neither harming nor being harmed

- Awareness of your connectedness with nature
- Feeling grounded—comfort and security within your surroundings
- Respect and appreciation for your home, the Earth, and all of her inhabitants
- Contact with the Earth; breathing healthy air; drinking pure water; eating uncontaminated food; exposure to the sun, fire, or candlelight; immersion in warm water (all on a daily basis).

HOLISTIC MEDICAL TREATMENT AND PREVENTION

To begin to restore your body to a heightened state of harmony and to correct the present imbalance manifested by arthritic joints, your *primary goals* are:

(1) **To stop the degeneration of the cartilage and regenerate new cartilage**
(2) **To strengthen your immune system**
(3) **To address each of the possible causes of your arthritis.**

In meeting these goals, you can potentially cure your arthritis while you're healing your life. The word *cure* refers to a physical problem, while *heal* has to do with the condition of your life. It is, however, possible to cure your arthritic joints but still live an imbalanced life; or, conversely, you may feel whole, balanced, at peace with your life, while still experiencing some degree of joint pain. In essence, *this holistic approach will provide you with the potential to do both—cure arthritis and heal your life—while you are engaged in the process of loving and nurturing your diseased joints along with the rest of you.*

Think of the Arthritis Survival Program as *a personalized course in self-healing and optimal well-being.* In this and the following chapters, you will be provided with a "curriculum" or, if you prefer, a "prescription" for improving six components of health while treating each of the primary causes of osteoarthritis. I have tried to simplify each component and have suggested "exercises" to help you find your own path to a greater level of physical, environmental, mental, emotional, spiritual, and social fitness. These exercises must be practiced regularly in order to be effective. (However, if after giving it a fair trial, a particular exercise feels too uncomfortable to you, then stop.) If you are willing to be patient—remember, it took years for you to develop your current state of health—I promise that you will feel better, although I cannot guarantee you will cure your arthritis. But your chances for doing so are far greater using this approach, especially if there is no major joint degeneration, than if you strictly adhered to the conventional medical treatment, which treats only symptoms. Holistic medicine is not an alternative but a complement to what you are already doing for your arthritis. It is also the most therapeutically sound and cost-effective approach to the treatment of chronic disease that I've found in nearly thirty years of practicing medicine. By taking responsibility for your own health, you become not only your own healer but a highly skilled practitioner of preventive medicine. You'll learn what *causes* your joints to ache and what relieves the pain, and will be able to make well-informed choices regarding your arthritic condition. You're also a pioneer of sorts, since the holistic self-care model presented on the following pages will soon become an essential part of the foundation of primary-care medicine. Keep in mind that although this is a course with a lot of homework, there are no exams or grades, no mistakes or failures; just a series of valuable lessons to help you feel more fully alive. Enjoy yourself! What do you have to lose?

Symptom Treatment

I would recommend beginning the Arthritis Survival Program with an aggressive approach to treating the symptoms of your arthritis. This includes consulting with your physician and making sure that you have treated your condition with the best methods that conventional medicine has to offer, even if they provide only temporary and symptomatic relief. It is also essential that you determine if the benefits of that treatment outweigh the liabilities. For instance, analgesics and anti-inflammatories may be harmful to the gastrointestinal tract, possibly causing stomach ulcers. If you've decided the risks of continuing this course of symptom treatment are too great or that it's not giving you effective relief, there are several options that will be offered to you in this chapter.

As you begin the Arthritis Survival Program, it is helpful to rate each of your symptoms on a scale of 1 to 10, with 1 being an almost incapacitating symptom and 10 being perfectly normal (no symptom). You can use the Symptom Chart (pages 29–30) and rate yourself at the end of each week. It provides you with both an objective (most of the symptoms can be measured objectively—you can either see, hear, or feel them) and a subjective (energy level, emotions) means of monitoring your progress. You don't need anyone else or an X ray or lab test to tell you how well you're doing. Please add any symptoms to this chart that are not listed but that often cause you discomfort.

The foundation of the physical aspect of holistic medical treatment is to love and nurture your body with safe, gentle, and effective therapies. You should have a much better idea of how to do that, especially for your arthritic joints, after reading this chapter. Remember that the essentials of the physical-health component of the Arthritis Survival Program can also be found in Chapter 1. As you begin, you should now keep in mind the image of a smooth, slippery, firm, radiant white, glistening cartilaginous surface inside your painful joint. (If mental imagery is difficult for you, then visualize the cartilaginous surface at the end of a chicken bone.) This healing vision can be expanded in any way you'd like. But it is important to keep it in mind as often as you can, since it will help you to stay focused on the goal of your treatment and, even more importantly, to make that *vision become a reality.*

TABLE 4.1

Symptom Chart

Began Arthritis Survival Program on _____ .
Rate symptoms from 1 (worst) to 10 (best = normal).

SYMPTOM	BEGIN (date)	END WEEK 1	END WEEK 2	END WEEK 3	END WEEK 4	END WEEK 5	END WEEK 6	END WEEK 7	END WEEK 8	END WEEK 9	END WEEK 10	END WEEK 11	END WEEK 12
Pain													
Stiffness/range of motion													
Cracking													
Swelling													
Energy level/ stamina													
Strength													
Irritability													
Sleep quality													
Depression													
Weather tolerance (hot/cold)													
Other symptoms:													

MEDICATIONS (pharmaceutical drugs: Use a "✓" if still taking.)

VITAMINS/HERBS/SUPPLEMENTS (Use a "✓" if still taking.)

	BEGIN ___(date)	END WEEK 1	END WEEK 2	END WEEK 3	END WEEK 4	END WEEK 5	END WEEK 6	END WEEK 7	END WEEK 8	END WEEK 9	END WEEK 10	END WEEK 11	END WEEK 12

Physical Health Recommendations for Arthritis

Arthritis, like any other chronic condition viewed from a holistic medical perspective, is a systemic dis-ease reflecting an imbalance and disharmony in the whole person—body, mind, and spirit. However, if your initial treatment is aggressively directed toward healing and restoring balance to the arthritic joint, and subsequently your mental and spiritual health, and there is no major joint degeneration, you have an excellent chance of curing your arthritis using this holistic approach.

The first and foremost goal of treatment is to **stop the degeneration of cartilage and regenerate new cartilage.** In holistic medicine this objective equates to the physical response to nurturing the dysfunctional joint. Physiologically, every organ, tissue, and body part functions more efficiently with a maximal supply of oxygen—our body's most critical nutrient—along with the other essential nutrients. Since oxygen and the other essential nutrients are transported through the blood, and blood consists almost entirely of water, anything that *enhances* *blood flow* to the painful joint—e.g., increased water intake, exercise, massage and body work, healing touch, breathing exercises, physical therapy—should improve the arthritic condition. Although cartilage itself has no direct blood supply and is nourished through an exchange of nutrients through the synovial fluid, it does derive indirect benefit from improved blood flow to the joint. *Relieving stress on the joint* (e.g., losing weight, reducing activity), *eliminating any food allergens or other triggers of inflammation of the cartilage,* and *taking supplements that support the growth of new cartilage* are also methods of directly **strengthening, healing, and loving your joints.**

Diet

The first step in treating arthritis is to *remove all inflammatory causes.* Researchers at the National Public Health Institute in Helsinki, Finland, have recently discovered that people drinking four or more cups of *coffee* a day are twice as likely to develop arthritis than occasional drinkers. Anyone consuming eleven or more cups daily may be increasing their risk of arthritis by fifteen times. A relatively small proportion of people with arthritis have *food allergies* and sensitivities that cause joint inflammation. Dairy products, wheat, corn, citrus fruit, peanuts, and especially *nightshade plants* (including potatoes, peppers, eggplant, tomatoes, and tobacco) are the foods most often responsible for contributing to arthritis. The adverse effect from nightshades is not usually due to an allergic reaction but to a toxin called solanine. Eliminating nightshades from your diet for at least three months, and an allergy elimination diet as outlined in the Phase I of the *New Life Eating Plan®* (*NLEP*), a hypoallergenic diet (see below), eliminates dairy, wheat, and any other repetitively eaten food for at least three weeks. This helps to determine if food allergy is contributing to your arthritis; gradually re-introducing them (one new food every three to four days) will reveal to you which specific foods, if any, provoke symptoms.

The next step is to *remove or decrease consumption of most animal products other than fish and healthy eggs,* which will help to eliminate excess calcium, mineral deposits, and acid from the joints. The most effective way to do this is by following the New Life Eating Plan developed by Todd Nelson, N.D., a Denver naturopathic doctor and the co-author of this book. He has for many years experienced excellent outcomes with his nutritional approach to treating arthritis. By eating according to his diet, you are eliminating the common food allergens and increasing raw fruits and vegetables. The NLEP is unique because it is nutrient-dense, hypoallergenic, low-yeast, high in phytonutrients (e.g., berries, cherries, and green and yellow vegetables), high in essential fatty acids (see page 50), low in nightshades, and low in land-animal products. It helps in treating arthritis by:

- eliminating possible food allergens
- stabilizing insulin levels (Elevated insulin or low-insulin sensitivity can increase pro-inflammatory chemicals.)
- correcting leaky gut and dysbiosis (an imbalance of the bacterial flora in the bowel), often resulting from long-term use of non-steroidal anti-inflammatory drugs (NSAIDs). Leaky gut contributes to inflammation of the joint by recirculating large, undigested molecules that, in turn, trigger the inflammatory cascade of chemicals.

The following is Phase I of the NLEP, which, for best results, should be followed for a minimum of three months. Phase II of the NLEP, presented on page 97, expands your dietary choices to create and maintain a lifetime of exceptional eating.

New Life Eating Plan: Phase I

Nutrient-Dense, Hypoallergenic Diet for Arthritis

Vegetables
50–60 percent of total diet = 3 to 6 cups daily
High-water content vegetables
Raw or lightly steamed
Fresh, organic, clean

STEAMED OR STIR-FRIED IN WATER AND SPICES

Most gentle (great for initial detoxification or cleansing diet): zucchini, celery, green beans, spinach, parsley, crook-necked squash

If you have digestive problems then avoid the following vegetables for 3 weeks; if digestion is normal then include them in Phase I: steamed broccoli, cabbage, bok choy, chard, kale, cauliflower, collard greens, mustard greens, beet greens, cabbage.

RAW

Baby greens, celery, carrots, cucumber, jicama, snow peas, sprouts, grated beets, red leaf lettuce, romaine lettuce, Bibb lettuce, green leaf lettuce, broccoli, radishes.

Fruits

All organic fruits are acceptable except citrus, e.g., oranges, grapefruit; lemons are an exception. Emphasize berries and cherries. No bananas for 2 months.

Do not mix fruits with other foods; eat as snacks between meals.

Whole Grains

Sprouted or cooked like rice (see Grain Preparation Chart, page 36).

Organic, clean—available in bulk at health food stores

Only eat the non-gluten grains: brown rice, millet, quinoa, amaranth. Rotate grains every four days.

Tasty as breakfast cereals, in salads and soups, in casseroles and stir-fries (excellent for dinners).

Store away from light and heat in airtight containers. Combine with beans and legumes occasionally if tolerated.

Starchy Vegetables

Squashes

(Avoid potatoes: They're nightshades. If you want to try adding potatoes, use new red potatoes, sweet potatoes, or yams.)

Protein

Recommended: raw organic nuts (almonds, filberts, pecans) and seeds (sunflower, pumpkin, sesame, flax), raw organic nut butters (no peanuts)—sprouted or soaked overnight or ground (12 nuts or handful of seeds = 1 serving)

Deepwater ocean fish (perch, salmon, halibut, orange roughy, sole, cod), farm-fresh fertile eggs—free of chemical additives

UltraInflamX Medical Food (from Metagenics) under a physician's supervision

Soy: tofu, soy yogurt, soy milk, tempeh

Minimize organic red meat, poultry, and lamb.

(Vegetarians: Bean and grain combinations are recommended.)

Protein powders: whey, soy, or rice-based.

Flaxseed Oil

Do not heat or cook with flaxseed oil.

1 to 2 tablespoons daily or 2 capsules twice daily with food

On grains or vegetables

With protein meals

As a salad dressing

Keep refrigerated and away from light.

Use within 6 weeks of opening.

Other oils: extra virgin olive oil: in salads, stir-fries, cooking; canola oil: in baking

Pure Water

Eight 8-oz glasses (or ½ oz/lb of body weight) daily between meals. (Allow only 2 to 4 oz. with a meal.)

Beverages

Fresh carrot, celery, or beet juice, or green drink—diluted 30 to 50 percent

Fresh fruit juices (not citrus)—diluted 70 percent

Herb teas (not citrus).

Suggestions for Implementing the Diet

(1) After shopping, chop up and store vegetables in separate containers for quick and easy use in stir-fries, salads, soups, and snacks.

(2) Cook 2 to 3 grains at once at the beginning of the week for convenient use as breakfast hot cereals, in salads, stir-

fries, soups, and casseroles. Cooked grains will last 5 or more days in the refrigerator and can be frozen as well.

(3) Prepare a couple of healthy sauces or dressings ahead of time for easy meals with already chopped vegetables and prepared grains.

(4) Prepare large meals with plenty of leftovers for easy lunches and snacks. Freeze leftovers for future meals.

(5) Use a Crock-Pot for soups, stews, chilies, and beans.

(6) Save vegetable stock when steaming vegetables for later use in sauces and soups. You can freeze the stock too.

(7) Keep your kitchen stocked with staples and foods from your favorite recipes.

(8) Freeze fruit such as bananas, blueberries, and grapes for snacks or use in smoothies.

(9) Take a water bottle with you wherever you go.

(10) Keep healthy snacks in your car and at work so you have healthy foods available when you get hungry.

Weight reduction, which is also strongly recommended in treating arthritis, should naturally occur when the NLEP and an exercise program are consistently practiced. In addition to food allergy assessment through an allergy elimination diet, food allergy testing is available through Great Smokies Laboratory in Asheville, NC (see Resource Guide).

MENU SUGGESTIONS FOR THE NEW LIFE EATING PLAN: PHASE I

Breakfast Suggestions

Non-gluten whole grain porridge (Recipe available at health food store.)

Non-gluten whole grain hot cereal (Recipe available at health food store.)

Mochi waffle

½ baked acorn squash

Nut butters

Baked sweet potatoes

12 raw almonds, walnuts, filberts, pecans, or pinenuts

TABLE 4.2

Grain Preparation Chart

Grain	Grain Family	Gluten	Appearance (dry)	Uses
Amaranth	amaranthus	NO	tiny, round, light colored, speckled with black grain	in porridge, pancakes, vegetable dishes; ground as flour; used in baking
Barley	cereal grass	YES	oblong, light colored with a lengthwise "crease"	in salads, vegetable dishes, soups; ground as flour
Buckwheat	sorrel	NO	groats—golden green, triangular shaped: kasha— toasted groats, golden brown	in salads, vegetable dishes; ground as flour
Corn	cereal grass	NO	polenta—coarsely stone-ground corn meal, yellow and brown	in porridge, cornbread, hominy, tortillas
Millet	cereal grass	NO	small, round, lemon-tasting, yellow color	in salads, vegetable dishes, puddings, porridge
Oats	cereal grass	YES	groats—long, slender, flake light brown	in porridge, salads; ground as flour
Quinoa	goosefoot	NO	white/brown, small discs	in salads, vegetable dishes
Rice	cereal grass	NO	oblong, light-colored varieties	in salads, vegetable dishes, puddings; ground as flour
Rye	cereal grass	YES	oblong, slender, grey/brown color	sprouting, in salads, vegetable dishes, bread
Triticale	cereal grass	YES	large, plump red/ brown	sprouting, in salads; ground as flour
Wheat	cereal grass	YES	soft wheat—plump, oblong, slight brown color; hard wheat— small, oblong, brown	sprouting, in salads, vegetable dishes; ground as flour

Water	Cook	Yield	Comments
2 cups	20 min	1 cup	Very high in protein; slightly sticky texture.
3 cups	1 hr 15 min	3½ cups	Always barley "pot" barley, not refined "pearl."
2 cups	15–20 min	2½ cups	Chewy or soft, depending on the amount of water used.
4 cups	25 min	3 cups	Look for "stone ground" to avoid rancid oils.
3 cups	30–45 min	3½ cups	If bitter in taste, strain off initial cooking water and add new boiling water.
1½ cups	30 min	2½ cups	Large flake oatmeal is processed; occasional use is fine.
2 cups	15 min	3 cups	Pronounced "keen-wa"; very high in protein.
2 cups	45 min	3 cups	Many varieties; try short, or long grains; buy organic.
3 cups	1 hour	2½ cups	Stronger, heartier flavor than wheat with less gluten.
3 cups	30–60 min	2⅔ cups	Cross between rye and wheat.
3 cups	2 hrs	2⅔ cups	Bulgur, cracked wheat, and couscous are processed; use occasionally.

Note: If grains are pre-soaked, drain the soaking water, decrease cooking water by ½ cup, and decrease cooking time by 5 to 15 minutes.

Breakfast Suggestions continued
Small handful of raw sunflower seeds or pumpkin seeds
Ground raw sesame or flaxseeds sprinkled on hot cereal
Nut butter or nut milk
Steamed vegetables
Eggs and vegetables: omelette or basted with steamed veggies
Protein Smoothie i.e., 4 oz plain soy milk, 4 oz water, soy or rice
     protein powder, ½–1 cup organic berries or cherries, ice
     cubes, blend

Lunch Suggestions
(Protein/vegetable combinations)
Fresh green salad with raw nuts or seeds
Fresh green salad with turkey, fish, lamb, beef, or chicken
Fresh green salad with sprouted beans or cooked beans
Steamed vegetables sprinkled with ground-up raw nuts or seeds
Steamed vegetables and an animal protein
Steamed vegetables or salad and bean, lentil, or pea soup
Vegetable and nut stir-fry (no rice)
Vegetable and animal protein stir-fry (no rice)
Fresh tuna salad with no mayonnaise
Vegetable and animal protein soup
Vegetable and bean soup
Vegetable soup or stew
Fresh vegetable sticks and nut butter for dip
Fresh vegetables and hummus for dip
Steamed asparagus wrapped in thinly sliced turkey breast
Turkey or chicken drumsticks and vegetables.

Dinner Suggestions
*(Complex carbohydrate/vegetable combinations. Protein foods may also
     be added)*
Vegetable and non-gluten whole-grain casserole
Vegetable and non-gluten whole-grain salad
Vegetable and non-gluten whole-grain soup
Vegetable nori rolls with no mustard
Steamed vegetables or green salad with new red potatoes
Vegetables and baked squash or sweet potatoes

Vegetables with beans and rice
Vegetable stir-fry with a non-gluten whole grain
Non-gluten pasta salad
Non-gluten pasta with dairy-free pesto sauce and vegetables
Dairy-free new red potato salad with vegetables
Vegetable sandwich on a non-gluten whole grain bread.*

Beverages
Herb teas, non-citrus
Fresh, organic vegetable juice diluted 50 percent
Pure water
Fresh grated ginger-root tea

Flavorings
Flaxseed oil for salad dressings or in place of butter on steamed
    vegetables or cooked grains
Cold-pressed olive oil or sesame oil (Omega Nutrition)
Braggs Liquid Aminos
Fresh lemon or lime in dressings or on steamed vegetables
Fresh herbs: cilantro, mint, basil, dill, parsley, or rosemary to fla-
    vor salads and grains
Fresh spices (see page 44) (Avoid salt and black pepper.)
Use Ghee instead of margarine or butter
Garlic (great for candida diets)
Ginger root
Nut butters for sauces and dressings

ALLERGY–FREE TREATS

Fresh organic fruit
Organic vegetable sticks
Raw organic almonds
Raw organic walnuts
Raw organic filberts
Raw organic pinenuts
Raw organic sunflower seeds

*Sauce and dressing recipes included on page 43.

Raw organic pumpkin seeds
Rye crackers with raw nut butters
Smoothies
Nut milks or nut cheeses
Fresh juices (dilute 1:1 with water)
Juice popsicles
Frozen fruit popsicles
Applesauce or other fruit sauce
Baked apples
Steamed fruit
Fruit salad
Agar-agar and fruit juice mixed
Rice or millet pudding
Non-gluten or whole grain muffins
Non-gluten or whole grain pasta
Carrot/raisin/apple/celery salad
Hummus
Leftovers
Nori roll

SAMPLE RECIPES TO INCLUDE IN THE NLEP: PHASE I
(For additional recipes, refer to the cookbook *Vital Abundance* by Karen Falbo.)

Breakfast recipes

WHOLE GRAIN PORRIDGE

Use leftover (already cooked) non-gluten grains: brown rice, millet, amaranth, or quinoa. Place the cold grain in the blender with water, juice, rice milk, or nut milk. The amount of liquid will determine how thick the porridge will be. Blend together to desired consistency. Heat the porridge. Add pure maple syrup and flaxseed oil to taste. Be creative and try other flavorings such as cinnamon, almond butter, banana, ground flaxseeds, apple sauce, or almond slivers. No two porridges are alike. (For candida diets, do not include fruit or sweeteners unless advised otherwise.)

WHOLE GRAIN HOT CEREAL

If you like Cream of Wheat, why not try "cream of millet," "cream of amaranth," or "cream of quinoa." Pick any non-gluten grain and grind up ½ cup in a coffee grinder.

Add the grain very gradually to 1½ cups boiling water or apple juice, stirring constantly. Simmer for 5 minutes. Top it off with maple syrup, nutmilk, and flax oil. Also try nuts and seeds, cinnamon, apple sauce, or banana slices. It's quick, easy, and yummy! (For candida diets, do not add fruit or sweeteners unless advised otherwise.)

NUTMILK

Place ½ cup raw almonds, sunflower seeds, or sesame seeds, 1 tablespoon maple syrup or honey (optional), and two cups of water in the blender. Blend until smooth and creamy. Strain milk through a cheesecloth. Flavor with cinnamon or pure vanilla. It's delicious hot or cold and a great milk substitute for baking.

SPROUTED GRAINS

Soak a non-gluten grains for 12 to 24 hours, rinsing twice daily until a tiny ¼-inch sprout begins to appear. At this point, spread the sprouts out on a towel and allow them to dry for 1 to 4 hours. Do not allow them to wither and harden. Place in refrigerator and they will last 3 to 10 days. To serve, warm the sprouts very carefully in a pan with melted butter or soak in hot tap water for a minute or so. Eat them for breakfast or in place of cooked grains at other meals. Sprouts are high in fiber, the enzymes in the grains have not been destroyed by heat, and they are often less allergenic than cooked grains.

ACORN SQUASH

Cut squash in half and steam facedown for 20 to 30 minutes. Set on oven dish and fill with 1 teaspoon butter and 1 teaspoon honey or maple syrup. Place in 350-degree oven for 10 minutes. Also delicious with flaxseed oil, but do not add until after baking. (For candida diets, avoid maple syrup or honey.)

Lunch and/or Dinner Recipes

BIELER'S BROTH

Steam 2 medium-size zucchini, a handful of green beans, and 2 stalks of celery until they are very soft. Place the vegetables and the steaming water in the blender and blend for 1 to 2 minutes until smooth. Add fresh parsley and serve hot.

VEGETABLE SOUP

In a large saucepan, sauté diced celery, carrot, zucchini, broccoli, cauliflower, cabbage, onion, and garlic in a little pure water. Cover with water and add 1 tablespoon oregano, 1 tablespoon basil, and cayenne to taste. Simmer ½ hour. Serve, then add Bragg's Liquid Aminos to taste. Also try this soup with diced new red potatoes or sweet potatoes.

SPLIT PEA SOUP

Dice and sauté carrots, celery, and onions. Boil 1 cup green split peas in ½ to 1 quart water. Add vegetables after 20 minutes. Add ¼ teaspoon thyme.

CLEAN CASSEROLE

Steam zucchini and celery for 5 minutes. Turn off burner, add a good portion of mung bean sprouts, and let sit for 5 minutes. Place ½ inch of cooked rice in bottom of buttered casserole dish. Pour vegetables on top of rice and sprinkle with sunflower seeds. Bake at 350 degrees for 20 minutes. Allow to cool slightly, then add 1 to 2 tablespoons of ghee or flaxseed oil, and sprinkle with Bragg's Liquid Aminos.

CURRY RICE

Sauté mushrooms and onions in ghee. Add cooked brown rice, a little tamari and 2 tablespoons curry powder. Garnish with fresh chopped parsley. Serve with sautéed vegetables, and a side of raisins and/or coconut.

QUINOA SALAD

1 cup quinoa, rinsed 2 to 3 times, 1¾ cups pure water, ½ cup finely diced cucumber or 4 celery stems, finely diced green

onion, ¼ cup finely diced fresh cilantro, ⅓ cup corn kernels, 3 tablespoons fresh lime juice, 2 tablespoons sesame oil, 2 tablespoons flaxseed oil, sea salt to taste, 1 teaspoon rice syrup or honey (optional).

Bring water to a boil in a 1 quart pot, then add quinoa. Reduce heat and simmer, covered, for 15 minutes, stirring occasionally until grain is tender. Remove from heat and let cool, uncovered. Toss cucumber, green onion, cilantro, and corn kernels with cooked quinoa. Combine the lime juice, oils, salt, cayenne, and honey and add to quinoa. Stir thoroughly with a fork to coat the grains and vegetables.

VEGGIE SANDWICH

Pile high on a non-gluten bread, any or all of the following: grated carrot, cucumber, green pepper, onion, sprouts, lettuce, avocado. Sprinkle with your favorite herbs and spices.

ROSE'S SAUCE

Mix together 1 to 2 tablespoons flaxseed oil, 1 to 2 tablespoons raw sesame tahini, 2 teaspoons Bragg's Liquid Aminos, and fresh lemon juice to taste. Top with steamed vegetables (cabbage, onion, zucchini, and red peppers make a great combination) and wild rice. Serve hot. This also makes a great salad dressing if you decrease the tahini and increase the lemon juice. Add your favorite herbs and spices.

Non-Dairy Salad Dressing

¾ cup	(180ml)	Omega brand flaxseed oil*
¼ cup	(60ml)	apple cider vinegar
1 tsp	(5ml)	Dijon mustard
1 tsp	(5ml)	Bragg Liquid Aminos
3 to 5 cloves		garlic (crushed)
6 drops		Tabasco sauce
1 Tbsp	(15ml)	sweet basil

*Certified organic by Farm Verified Organic (FVO) and Organic Crop Improvement Association (OCIA).

½ tsp	(2ml)	tarragon
½ tsp	(2ml)	oregano
1 tsp	(5ml)	maple syrup (optional)
1 Tbsp	(15ml)	capers

Blend in blender or food processor. Store leftover dressing in the fridge. The dressing will keep for several days. Add extra garlic if you like!

Spices and Herbs

Purchase a wide variety of whole, real, unadulterated herbs and seasonings (at your local health food store), grind them if they have not been already, and put them in salt and pepperlike dispensers for ready use.

Seasonings (spices and herbs) should enhance the natural flavor of your food. Carefully note the aroma of your food and then note the aroma of the various herbs that you have on hand. Let your intuition decide which herbs or combination of herbs to use, then proceed to do so sparingly to see if your palate is in agreement with your olfaction (smell).

Add some international flair to your cooking. With the right seasoning and your imagination, you can create any flavor you wish!

Middle Eastern—garlic, onion, turmeric, cinnamon, cumin, cloves, cayenne, mint

Hungarian—onion, garlic, paprika, caraway, dill, white pepper

Mexican—garlic, onion, fresh chilies, oregano, cumin, allspice, cinnamon, cilantro

Italian—onion, garlic, basil, oregano, rosemary, marjoram, red pepper, bay leaf

Indian—garlic, ginger root, onion, coriander, paprika, cumin, turmeric, cayenne, mint

French—garlic, onion, thyme, rosemary, bay leaf

Chinese—garlic, ginger root, cayenne; add hoison or tamari sauce, sesame or peanut oil, and rice-wine vinegar for additional flavor.

Fasting, or Detoxification

Periodic supervised *fasting,* also known as *detoxification,* has had a very high success rate in reducing or eliminating joint pain for the past century in Europe. Many of the clinics throughout Europe have had remarkable results with periodic juice fasting. Gabriel Cousens, M.D., at his Tree of Life Rejuvenation Center in Patagonia, Arizona, has administered a *juice fasting* program for treating arthritis to a large number of people and has been consistently successful. Fasting enhances the eliminative and cleansing capacity of the lungs, skin, liver, and kidneys. It also rests and restores the digestive system and helps to relax the nervous system and mind. If you're considering fasting as a therapeutic option, it is best to do it under the supervision of a well-trained physician. Dr. Nelson frequently uses the product UltraInflamX Medical Food (Metagenics—available only to physicians) along with a cleansing diet.

Vitamins, Minerals, and Supplements

In this section most of the products we recommend are available in health food stores and some are only available through Thriving Health Products. You can refer to the Product Index on page 207 for information on how you can obtain them.

Glucosamine sulfate is a naturally occurring building block of the substances (both proteoglycans and collagen) that make up cartilage. It is primarily produced in the body. As a dietary supplement it is revolutionizing the treatment of arthritis. It has the proven capability of both regenerating cartilage and inhibiting cartilage-degrading enzymes, thereby *slowing or preventing continued deterioration, while relieving joint pain and improving mobility.* Although it is not an anti-inflammatory, a multitude of studies (nearly 300, including 20 double-blind studies) have shown that glucosamine can also effectively relieve the pain of osteoarthritis as well as NSAIDs and with little or no side effects. One eight-week study compared the effects of glucosamine to ibuprofen. While the ibuprofen seemed to be working a bit better during the first two weeks and its benefits remained stable after that, those taking glucosamine continued to gradually improve throughout the remainder of the eight weeks.

The use of glucosamine for treating arthritis was first reported by German physicians in 1969, and for many years it has been approved for this use in a number of European countries. American veterinarians have been using it successfully on dogs and horses. On March 14, 2000, the American Medical Association (AMA) issued a news release describing a meta-analysis published in *The Journal of the AMA* (JAMA), which concludes that glucosamine and chondroitin supplements may have moderate to large therapeutic effects on osteoarthritis of the knee and hip. One landmark study, in which biopsies of arthritic knees were taken before and after thirty days of glucosamine sulfate therapy, dispels the commonly held belief that arthritis is an irreversible disease. The results showed that the degenerating cartilage had been replaced by much healthier cartilage.

This supplement is considered safe, but it can occasionally produce heartburn and diarrhea. This is probably because it is a difficult substance to digest, which is why it should be taken with meals. This will usually minimize or prevent a possible upset stomach. When capsules are ingested this way, about 90 percent of the glucosamine is absorbed into your body. Glucosamine promotes the healing of joints rather than merely relieving symptoms, and as a result it may take two to four weeks for pain relief, and four to twelve weeks to experience maximum benefit. It is available in most health food stores. The recommended therapeutic dosage is 1,000mg three times per day for twelve weeks, followed by a maintenance dosage of 500mg, three times per day with meals (or 750mg twice a day). One study suggests that people taking a diuretic may need to take higher doses of the glucosamine to get its full effect. There are no known drug interactions, but there is some concern for diabetics (from animal studies) that it may raise blood sugar levels. The highest-quality brands of glucosamine sulfate that I am familiar with are available through Thriving Health Products and

Enzymatic Therapy, both of which are available in selected health food stores.

Chondroitin sulfate is another naturally occurring component of joint cartilage. The body uses glucosamine to help make chondroitin. Although not as numerous as for glucosamine, there are several impressive studies documenting the therapeutic benefits of chondroitin for arthritis. In 1998, the journal *Osteoarthritis and Cartilage* published three double-blind placebo-controlled studies that documented the effectiveness of chondroitin sulfate in treating arthritis. It is widely used in Europe primarily in an injectable form, which is injected directly into arthritic joints. This form of chondroitin is not readily available in the U.S. Like glucosamine, *oral chondroitin sulfate can significantly reduce the pain and slow the progressive deterioration of the joints* in people suffering with arthritis. As you've already learned, there is no conventional treatment for arthritis that protects the joints and prevents them from worsening. It helps provide the body with the building blocks it needs to repair itself, and it also is believed to inhibit the activity of the enzymes that break down cartilage. Chondroitin works slowly, with improvement usually noted after three months and progressing up to one year or more. It is usually taken in combination with glucosamine. The recommended dosage is 400mg three times per day. Since chondroitin is difficult to digest, it should be taken with meals and with digestive enzymes (described below). I recommend Thriving Health's Glucosamine Intensive Care as a high-quality joint supplement combining glucosamine and chondroitin sulfate.

The best natural source of the cartilage-building sulfates is *bovine (cow) cartilage.* However, most companies that process this cartilage do so unnaturally, using caustic solvents like the acetone in nail polish remover. The majority also use heat to prepare the cartilage for processing, which can kill the nutrients. It is best to take glucosamine or chondroitin, that has been made from bovine cartilage processed without the use of chemicals or heat.

It is also important to take digestive enzymes, such as *brome-*

lain (found in pineapple), *papain* (found in papaya), *chymotrypsin,* and *pancreatin* along with the above-mentioned sulfates to improve their digestion and absorption, hence improving their benefits. The enzymes can also reduce lymph congestion, toxicity, and tissue inflammation. Raw food enzymes, such as those found in the Metagenics product SpectraZyme (only available from health professionals), have also been effective in reducing food allergen antigens in the gut, which may contribute to inflammation in the joints. Digestive enzymes are readily available in most health food stores.

The supplement *S-adenosylmethionine* (*SAMe*) has been successfully used for treating arthritis in Europe for over twenty years, but has only recently become available in the U.S. Numerous studies have documented its effectiveness for treating arthritis. Due to some controversy regarding its purity, it is preferable to use SAMe as the pharmaceutical-grade finished product that is imported in tablet form from Europe, rather than other preparations that are currently being sold in the U.S. The European tablets are more expensive but chemically stabilized so they will not decompose rapidly. It has also been used for treating depression and strengthening the liver. SAMe is produced by every cell in the body and is part of a biochemical process that helps to regulate hormones and mood-altering neurotransmitters. It contributes to the production of the amino acids cysteine and taurine, and the potent antioxidant glutathione. Blood levels of this substance are low in people with arthritis. (It may be contraindicated in people with elevated homocysteine levels.)

Since it was first discovered by Italian chemists in 1952, most of the research on SAMe has been performed in that country. An Italian survey of studies published in 1987 found that SAMe was almost as effective as ibuprofen in relieving arthritis symptoms, without the potential for harmful gastrointestinal side effects. One of the best studies compared SAMe to naproxen (Aleve and Naprosyn) 750mg per day and found that it provided as much pain relief. However, naproxen worked more quickly (within two weeks) and produced more side effects (digestive upset), while the full effect of SAMe was not apparent until four weeks. In another double-blind comparative study, SAMe was found to be as effective in treating arthritis as the drug piroxicam (Feldene).

In addition to relieving inflammation, there is some evidence that SAMe, like glucosamine and chondroitin, can regenerate cartilage. Its benefits have been found to continue for months after treatment is stopped. One animal study suggests that it may even help protect joints from developing arthritis. The dosage is 400mg three times per day for twenty-one days or until symptoms improve. Then reduce to 200mg one to three times per day to keep symptoms under control. It is quite safe, with possible minimal stomach distress. A positive side effect of SAMe is that it can act as an effective antidepressant. Since many people suffering the chronic pain of arthritis may also be depressed, this is obviously a desirable effect. However, SAMe should not be combined with antidepressant medications. Another positive benefit is that it seems to have a protective effect upon the lining of the stomach, and it may also protect the liver from damage caused by alcohol and other liver toxins. The major drawback of taking SAMe is the expense. A full dosage of 1,200mg daily can cost hundreds of dollars a month.

Methylsulfonylmethane (MSM) is a good source of sulfur, which can be used to build glycosaminoglycans, a key ingredient of collagen (needed for cartilage) and synovial fluid in the joints. In recent years there are many people who claim to have experienced a marked improvement in their arthritis through the daily use of this supplement. MSM is not scientifically proven to treat arthritis. Yet, the widespread anecdotal evidence of its use has attracted a great deal of media attention. In their compelling book *The Miracle of MSM,* Drs. Jacob, Lawrence, and Zucker present the history, theory, and use of this product. It appears very safe and is reported to help arthritis by reducing pain, decreasing inflammation, assisting in joint repair, relieving muscle spasm, increasing blood flow throughout the body, lessening scar tissue, slowing degeneration of cartilage, and supplying biologically active sulfur compounds. From their clinical experience in treating thousands of patients, they recommend a maintenance dosage of 2,000mg per day. Those individuals with more severe pain should gradually increase the dose by a gram (1,000mg) every week, or to bowel tolerance. This can be as much as 8 to 10 grams per day in a crystalline form that can be dissolved in water. They have patients taking up to 40 to 65 grams per day safely, but only under medical supervision. MSM appears to be a promising therapy that still needs additional clinical and scientific data to support it.

There are a wide variety of *collagen* supplements available at health food stores, in addition to Thriving Health's Collagen Support.

Essential fatty acids (EFAs) in the form of *omega-3* oils, EPA/DHA, from cold-water fish (salmon, sardines, and tuna; see page 92) and *flaxseed* oil (contains almost twice as much omega-3 as do fish oils), have been shown to significantly improve the symptoms of arthritis, primarily by inhibiting the process of cartilage destruction. The most effective way to take omega-3 oils is in the form of *EPA* (eicosapentaenoic acid) in a dosage of up to 600mg four times per day for twelve weeks, then reduce to three times per day; *DHA* (docosahexaenoic acid), up to 400mg four times a day for two months, then reduce to three times per day; and *flaxseed* oil, one tablespoon twice per day with meals or three capsules 1,000mg each, two times per day with meals. There are many varieties of EFAs available in health food stores containing EPA and DHA. However, you'll need to check the amounts of each of the oils to be sure you're taking the proper dosage. Thriving Health's Super Potency Essential Fatty Acids provides the recommended dosage.

Calcium is a strong contributor to cartilage health and in helping to maintain bone density. Calcium, in an MCHA form, is recommended 400 to 600mg 3 times per day. Thriving Health's Calcium Supreme is a high quality calcium containing glucosamine.

Niacinamide, or *vitamin B$_3$,* is one of the oldest and most successful treatments for arthritis. It was first described in the 1940's by Dr. William Kaufman, who observed improvement in joint range-of-motion, pain, and swelling in patients with arthritis.

Improvement was usually noted after three to four weeks of treatment, with a usual dose of 250mg six times a day. More recently, Wayne Jonas, M.D., former chairman of the NIH Department of Complementary/Alternative Medicine, published a study in 1996 in which niacinamide (500mg six times per day) was shown to significantly improve the severity of arthritis and joint mobility. The evidence indicates that niacinamide can be a valuable contributor to your program for superior joint protection. Niacinamide not only increases circulation into the joint spaces, it actually reduces chemicals that can accelerate cartilage damage. Very recent studies have found that free radicals can damage DNA which then activates certain enzymes, most notably one called PARS (poly ADP-ribose synthetase), that ultimately reduces cellular repair energy and can even end up causing premature cell death. An increase in PARS destabilizes joint integrity. Cartilage matrix production slows down and there is an increase in cartilage loss. Niacinamide effectively inhibits PARS production, as well as reduces chemicals called cytokines, (especially a cytokine called tumor necrosis factor alpha—TNFa), which are triggers for inflammation. Effective doses of niacinamide range from 1,000 to 3,000mg per day, and is best taken in small, frequent doses. For example, 500mg taken four times a day is more effective than 1,000mg twice a day. Niacinamide is relatively safe, but can in rare instances cause liver damage. For this reason it is recommended that if you are taking a dosage in excess of 1,500mg a day, a blood test for liver enzymes should be done after three months of treatment and annually thereafter. If liver enzymes are elevated, then reduce the dosage. Alan Gaby, M.D., a holistic physician who has been using high dosages of niacinamide with his arthritis patients for almost twenty years, is not aware of any instance of permanent liver damage. Dr. Gaby has also noted that some of his patients using niacinamide have reported significant improvement in mood, energy level, and overall well-being.

The *antioxidants* (substances that prevent oxidation of cell membranes and thereby prevent cell damage): *NAC* (*N-acetylcysteine*), 200 to 800mg per day to reduce the stress of oxidative damage to the joints, especially following aerobic exercise. Studies within the last couple of years show that NAC is a top performer as a powerful antioxidant. It provides a source of cysteine, an amino acid, that is a precursor to a protein called glutathione, (GSH). GSH is the principal factor in the body protecting us from free radical damage. Healthy cartilage and synovial fluid require antioxidant protection to continue to be well lubricated and flexible. NAC, like niacinamide, inhibits TNFa and therefore promotes collagen production. The Thriving Health product, Artho Extra, combines both niacinamide and NAC as an effective formula for reducing PARS and TNFa, and promoting joint repair and optimal function; *vitamin C,* 1,000 to 6,000mg per day in an ascorbate form or Ester-C (essential for collagen synthesis and connective tissue repair); *vitamin A* or beta-carotene 10,000 to 25,000 IU per day; and *vitamin E* 400 to 800 IU per day (has a mild anti-inflammatory effect and increases proteoglycans) have all demonstrated benefits in treating arthritis. The federal government's Institute of Medicine's recent (April 2000) guidelines on recommended daily dosages for vitamins suggests a maximum of 2,000mg per day of C. The primary risk mentioned for megadoses of vitamin C was diarrhea. Although the Arthritis Survival dosages may exceed these limits, using an ascorbate form of C or Ester-C reduces the possibility of these adverse side effects since they are much better tolerated in the bowel than ascorbic acid (most common form of vitamin C). If diarrhea does occur, you can simply reduce the dosage. I personally have been taking an average of 6,000mg of vitamin C daily for the past fifteen years without any problems whatsoever. In fact, I'm healthier than I've ever been and so are most of my patients, the majority of whom also exceed the recommended maximum daily dose of vitamin C. Linus Pauling, a two-time Nobel Prize winner who did much of the original research on the therapeutic benefits of vitamin C, took 10,000mg daily and died at the age of 93.

A *vitamin B complex* is recommended at 50 to 100mg daily, but especially important is vitamin B_6 (50 to 100mg daily) and folic acid (400mcg daily), which can reduce the harmful side-effects of anti-inflammatory medications. Proanthocyanidin, found in *grape-seed extract,* in a dosage of 100 to 300mg per day acts as a strong anti-inflammatory. Masquelier's OPC (the highest strength grape seed) is available through Arthritis Survival. The *minerals* selenium 200mcg per day (enhances the effectiveness of vitamin E); zinc arginate or glycinate, 30 to 50mg per day; copper aspirinate, 2mg per day (avoid taking it at the same time as zinc); magnesium, 500mg per day; and manganese, 30mg per day should also be taken daily. A recent study showed manganese in combination with glucosamine and chondroitin improved arthritic symptoms of the knee.

The following *amino acids* are also helpful: *methionine,* for cartilage support, 200 mg 3 times per day, has been shown in some studies to be more effective than ibuprofen in treating arthritis (methionine can be derived from SAMe, but do not take SAMe and methionine at the same time as it may supply excess methionine); *L-glutamine,* 5 grams twice a per day in powder form is best, for healing the intestinal lining of leaky gut. Amino acids are the building blocks of protein and it is important to include complete protein (not from land animals) in your daily diet three to four times per day. A protein powder from organic soy, lactalbumin, or rice can be added for additional protein in a smoothie.

Mixed *bioflavonoids* including quercetin, 500mg three times per day, are helpful in reducing inflammation and supporting connective tissue. AMNI makes an excellent bioflavanoid called Flavanall, which is available through holistic physicians.

Probiotics (products that help to restore normal bacterial flora to the bowel) consisting of *lactobacillus acidophilus* and *bifidobacterium,* are particularly helpful in cases of dysbiosis, candidiasis, and leaky gut. Low-grade bacterial infections such as *klebsiella pneumoniae* and parasitic infections like *blastocystis hominus* have been linked to an increase in arthritic pain due to their associated toxicity in the joints. Probiotics are effective in combating these low-grade infections in addition to healing a leaky gut. The dosage is ½ teaspoon or two capsules three times per day, preferably on an empty stomach. Buy only refrigerated brands that clearly state an expiration date between one and ten months from the date the item is purchased.

Herbs

- **Boswellia** *(Boswellia serrata)*—a gum resin found in certain trees in India that has a strong analgesic effect. The boswellic acids also provide a wide range of anti-inflammatory functions, reduce joint swelling, and increase blood supply to the joints, thus promoting healing. It has been researched and used extensively in India as an Ayurvedic (traditional Indian medical) treatment for arthritis. It can be combined with curcumin and bromelain. The dosage is 500mg standardized to 70 percent boswellic acids, three to five times per day between meals. Arthritis Survival's Herbal Joint Relief meets this standard and includes curcumin and ginger.
- **Curcumin** *(Curcuma longa)*—an extract of the common spice turmeric, it is an effective anti-inflammatory and antioxidant. It increases secretion of cortisol (the body's natural cortisone) and also sensitizes receptors for adrenal hormones, making these hormones more effective as anti-inflammatory agents. Curcumin also helps to prevent the release of leukotriene (a substance causing inflammation) from white blood cells. The recommended dosage is 400mg containing 95 percent curcuminoids three times per day between meals and combined with 1,000mg of bromelain.
- **Ginger** *(Zingiber officinale)*—acts as an anti-inflammatory and natural COX–2 inhibitor that is well supported by scientific studies. It is also a digestive aid that soothes and relaxes the intestinal tract. The dosage is 0.5 to 1mg of powdered ginger daily or as a tea—one grated teaspoon of fresh ginger in a cup of hot water, twice a day. More simply you may take a standardized extract (5% or more gingerol) of ginger combined with 500 to 1,000mg of mixed bioflavonoids or include it in your diet.

- **Cayenne** *(capsaicin)*—available as an OTC ointment or cream for analgesia (blocks substance P, present in arthritic joints) and for increasing circulation to the joint. Cayenne ointment should be rubbed into the skin of the affected joints three or four times per day for at least a week. It is also available as a capsule, with a dosage of 500mg three times per day.
- **Devil's claw** *(Harpagphytum procumbens)*—an analgesic and anti-inflammatory, 1 to 2 grams three times per day. A recent double-blind study from France found that Devil's claw, 6 capsules (435mg each) taken daily for four months significantly reduced pain and the use of NSAIDs and analgesics.
- **Hawthorn berry** *(Crataegus oxyacantha)*—contains flavonoids that have an anti-inflammatory effect and can also enhance the integrity and stability of the collagen matrix, one of the primary components of cartilage. It is best taken as an extract, ¼ to ½ teaspoon three times per day.
- **White willow bark or meadowsweet**—contains salicin, the same active ingredient found in aspirin, which makes it an effective analgesic, especially for acute pain. The dosage is a 4:1 standardized extract, ½ teaspoon of tincture or 2 capsules, 200 to 400mg three times per day between meals.
- **Licorice root** *(Glycyrrhiza glabra)*—an anti-inflammatory that can also inhibit estrogen activity if levels are too high. The higher incidence of arthritis among women suggests that estrogen may play a role in contributing to this condition. Licorice used long-term can elevate blood pressure and increase potassium loss. This herb is especially helpful in protecting your intestinal lining if you are taking non-steroidal anti-inflammatory medications. Effective doses of licorice root are ⅛ to ¼ teaspoon of a 5:1 solid extract up to three times per day (up to 1,000mg per day).
- **Yucca** *(Yucca schidigera)*—has long been used to reduce arthritic pain and especially stiffness. In the mid-1970s a study on 101 arthritic patients was performed at the National Arthritis Medical Clinic in Desert Hot Springs, CA. Of the fifty people in the study receiving an average of four yucca

tablets daily, 61 percent reported feeling less pain, stiffness, and swelling in their joints than did those on the placebo. The recommended dosage of yucca is four capsules twice a day on an empty stomach.

- **Celery seed extract** *(Apium graveolens)*—an essential oil in this seed acts like an antioxidant and reduces joint inflammation.
- **Castor oil hot packs**—apply to affected joint.
- **Super green foods**—helpful for extra alkalizing, for phytonutrient concentration, and for strengthening the immune system. Two excellent products are Pure Synergy and E-3.

Hydrotherapy

- Hot and cold showers to stimulate general circulation and act as a general tonic.
- Alternating hot and cold packs on the affected joint, or just cold packs.
- Hot Epsom salts baths or local bath or compress.

Hormones/Glandulars

Adrenal function is often compromised with osteoarthritis, and *adrenal* support is recommended. Adrenal testing through an Adrenal Stress Index is available through Great Smokies Lab or Diagnos-Techs Lab. I've used the product, Adrenal Complex, for many years with good results. Both *estrogen* and *progesterone* insufficiency may aggravate joint pain in women. If this is confirmed with lab tests (salivary hormone testing is especially accurate), then hormone replacement should be considered.

Exercise

The beneficial effects of exercise on arthritis were demonstrated in a 1997 study that appeared in JAMA. More than 430 adults, aged 60 or older, who considered themselves disabled by knee arthritis took part in exercise programs at medical schools in

Winston-Salem and Memphis. One group *walked* for forty minutes three times a week (warming up in advance, cooling down after); another group did **resistance training.** The program lasted eighteen months. People in both groups saw an 8-to-10-percent decrease in their disability level: Their pain lessened, their walking ability increased. (A control group, which did no exercise but simply got health education, did not get better). Although researchers used to be concerned that exercise could worsen arthritis, this and several other studies are proving the opposite is true.

Yoga and *tai chi* can be especially beneficial as part of the treatment program for arthritis. They both offer excellent range-of-motion exercise, which helps to relieve stiffness, restore flexibility, and help with joint movement. If you haven't already lost your full range of motion, exercises like these can help prevent such loss.

Whatever form of exercise you choose, it should not cause direct pounding or contribute to the deterioration of the affected joints. *Swimming* is also a good choice for arthritis sufferers.

Strength training is an important part of an arthritis exercise program, because weak muscles can contribute to joint problems. Many studies have shown that strength training can relieve knee pain while improving strength and physical functioning. Both *isometric exercise* (the muscle is contracted without moving the joint) and *isotonic exercise* (the joint is moved using elastic bands, weights, or resistance machines), can result in muscle strengthening. Isotonic exercise is a bit more effective. Water workouts can achieve similar results.

Aerobic exercise is also recommended for arthritis. Just as the aforementioned study demonstrated with walking, continuous movement for a minimum of ten minutes can definitely reduce pain and improve physical functioning. In addition to walking and swimming, other options for aerobic exercise include cycling (at low pedal resistance, over level surfaces at first), rowing, water walking, aqua aerobics, and ballroom or other low-impact dancing.

EXERCISE RECOMMENDATIONS
(IF YOU'RE JUST BEGINNING)

- **Exercise slowly and carefully.** Start with a modest amount and then increase. You may need instruction and coaching.
- **Gentle exercise should be a daily routine.** It's a long-term project—not something you do only occasionally.
- **Warm up before exercising.**
- **Heat can help.** If your joints are stiff, take a warm bath or shower just before exercising. Or apply a heating pad or hot pack to stiff joints.
- **Pick a time of day to exercise when you are least stiff and have less pain.** If you take pain relievers, take them one hour before exercising.
- **Avoid bouncing or high-impact exercise.** Stretch slowly.
- **Don't overdo exercise.** If you feel more pain than usual or sudden pain, then stop. If the pain persists, you've done too much. The advice of the trainer or physical therapist can be helpful in this case.

Professional Care Therapies

Arthritis Survival is a book and a holistic treatment program with a self-care orientation. However, there are situations in which therapies administered by a holistic physician or health practitioner are needed. For instance, if you have incorporated on a daily basis at least *three* of the above recommendations, and two of the three are dietary change and the recommended supplements, and you have experienced no improvement, then I'd suggest an appointment with a holistic physician. Most of you, however, will see a dramatic change in the condition of your arthritic joint(s). In that case, it is also perfectly acceptable and not uncommon for an individual to then choose to enhance the results of the Arthritis Survival Program with a complementary therapy administered by a physician or practitioner. A study that appeared in a September 1999 issue of the *Annals of Internal Medicine* revealed that 62 percent of patients with arthritis tried at least one type of complementary or alternative therapy. On average, patients had used 2.6 types. Of those who used a single method, 73 percent reported that chiropractors were helpful and 75 percent were helped by spiritual healers. (This includes hands-on healing methods such as healing touch and Reiki which are mentioned below under "Energy Medicine.")

The discipline of holistic medicine facilitates self-care while also including the prudent use of both conventional medicine and professional care alternatives. To my knowledge, the following modalities have all been effective in treating arthritis.

Osteopathic Medicine

As an osteopathic physician, the art and science of healing with which I'm most familiar is **osteopathic medicine,** which is essentially *holistic* medicine. It was founded and developed by Andrew Taylor Still, M.D., in 1874. The D.O. degree stands for Doctor of Osteopathic medicine, and D.O.'s are fully licensed physicians with unlimited rights and privileges to practice in all fifty states in the U.S. D.O.'s who have graduated from an osteopathic medical school have completed at a minimum a four-year undergraduate degree, four years of osteopathic medical education at one of the nineteen accredited osteopathic medical schools, and several years of residency training, depending upon their specialty and area of expertise. D.O.'s practice in all medical and surgical specialties, with the greatest percentage of practitioners being in primary care—family practice, pediatrics, and internal medicine.

A. T. Still was a fourth-generation M.D. who, after losing three of his own children one winter to an epidemic of meningitis, began to question the completeness of his medical training. He also suffered from terrible headaches for which he had found no solution in the medical model of his day. In the truly Hippocratic tradition, he became a seeker of answers to his own challenging medical problem. He became widely known for his effective, non-invasive, hands-on approach, and was referred to as a "bone-setter." Dr. Still was unsuccessful in his attempts to have his ideas and methods incorporated into the traditional medical model. Since his apprentices (seven-year apprenticeships were the accepted method of medical training in his day) were being taught medical "heresy," they were not granted the traditional M.D. degree. Instead, they were called D.O.'s—Doctors of Osteopathy. (The Latin root *osteo* means "bone," and *patheia* is Greek for "passion" or "suffering.")

When medical schools opened around the turn of the twentieth century, osteopathic students were still thought to be medical heretics, and thus began the two different forms of complete medical training, with two separate medical degrees—M.D. and D.O. Today, osteopathic medical schools have a very similar four-year curriculum to allopathic schools, with most of the same courses and textbooks but with several profound differences. Osteopathic medicine has at its core a holistic philosophy and a highly developed system of manual diagnostics and treatment techniques that are designed to stimulate our own innate healing and homeostatic mechanisms. The holistic principles upon which osteopathic medicine was founded are as follows:

(1) **A person is a complete dynamic unit of function, comprising body, mind, and spirit.** Osteopathic medicine recognizes the importance and uniqueness of each of these three elements in every individual and their relationship to disease and optimal health.

(2) **The body possesses self-regulatory mechanisms, which are self-healing in nature.** The primary objective of the osteopathic physician is to remove the obstacles to health, thereby enabling the body to seek its own path back toward health.

(3) **Structure and function are interrelated at all levels.** Therefore, if there is an asymmetry, restriction of motion, or tissue texture change present (these are called somatic dysfunctions by osteopathic physicians), one can predict a subsequent alteration in function of the same or referred regions.

(4) **Rational treatment is based on understanding and integrating the previous three principles.** Osteopathic medicine, in fact, offers a unique way of looking at

a patient and his disease. It is based upon a *whole person* perspective, an awareness that the body can heal itself and that its natural state is one of *optimal health,* combined with a scientific focus on understanding and treating the *causes of disease.*

Osteopathic manipulative treatment is as much an art as it is a science, and therefore each patient with arthritis may be treated a bit differently by an osteopathic physician. A thorough osteopathic structural exam from foot to head should precede any assumptions that all degenerative joint problems have their origins in the affected joint. This means that because of the interconnectedness of the body, the painful joint may manifest symptoms as a result of compensating for a primary structural problem elsewhere in the body that may be obstructing the flow of blood and nutrients into the synovial fluid. If other primary problem sites are not ruled out and/or diagnosed and treated appropriately, the arthritic joint may be treated repeatedly without significant improvement. This is often the case when one forgets that the body is a complete unit. Attempting to segment it often results in inadequate or unsuccessful treatment.

Osteopathic Manipulative Treatment (OMT) is highly effective for arthritis. OMT helps patients suffering from degenerative joint disease by promoting muscle and joint balance, increasing flexibility, decreasing pain, and normalizing blood and lymph flow. The types of OMT techniques most often used successfully for the treatment of arthritis are:

(1) **Low Velocity High Amplitude (LVHA),** which involves gently and slowly moving a patient's joints through as full a range of motion as possible. This encourages normalization of joint motion and muscle tension, promotes release of synovial fluid (enhancing joint nourishment and lubrication), and promotes normalization of blood and lymph flow.

(2) **Soft Tissue and Myofascial Release (ST/MFR),** which involves gentle and sometimes not-so-gentle ma-

nipulation of the muscles and the fascia which surrounds them, to promote balance and normalization of muscle tension. This promotes ease of movement, encourages improvement in posture, and promotes normalization of blood and lymph flow.

(3) **Facilitated Positional Release and Ligamentous Articular Release (FPR/LAR),** which involves gentle balancing of the muscles and ligaments supporting and influencing specific joints. These are extremely useful in tender and painful joints and are well tolerated when other techniques are not. When successfully performed, they result in marked pain relief and improvement in joint motion, which in turn promotes normalization of blood and lymph flow.

(4) **High Velocity Low Amplitude (HVLA),** which involves a rapid thrust through a very small range of motion. This is useful when there is a "locking" of a joint, since it helps to increase free motion and often will result in immediate pain relief. Care must be taken not to overuse this technique because it can potentially aggravate symptoms and cause inflammation.

(5) **Cranial osteopathy** (also known as *Osteopathy in the Cranial Field, or Craniosacral Therapy*), which is a system of diagnosis and treatment originally described and developed by William Garner Sutherland, D.O. He graduated from the American School of Osteopathy in 1900 and worked on developing what would become cranial osteopathy over the next fifty-plus years. His first publication on this subject was called the *Cranial Bowl* and was published in 1939. The underlying principles behind cranial osteopathy are the following:

(a) There is an inherent motion of the brain and spinal cord.

(b) There is regular fluctuation of the cerebrospinal fluid.

(c) There is inherent mobility of the intracranial and intraspinal membranes.

(d) There is articular mobility of the cranial bones.

(e) There is involuntary mobility of the sacrum between the hipbones.

A practitioner of cranial osteopathy evaluates and treats the entire body of the patient but is particularly good at diagnosing and addressing structural alterations in the head and sacrum (the bone at the base of the spine). This can be of significant benefit to an arthritis sufferer with a structural problem contributing to his joint pain. Cranial technique is usually gentle and rarely induces pain. There are intra-oral (fingers in your mouth) techniques as well as techniques that are performed on the outside of the head. The sacrum will be checked as well due to the strong connection between the sacrum and the skull via the dura mater (literally translated means "hard mother," it acts as a protective sheath covering the brain and spinal cord). Cranial manipulation can improve the way the joints function by eliminating obstruction, inflammation, and infection. Another very important benefit associated with cranial manipulation is that it tends to normalize autonomic nervous system imbalances. The autonomic nervous system is that part of the nervous system that controls "automatic" actions in the body, such as heart rate and breathing. It has been divided into a sympathetic and parasympathetic component—the sympathetic being associated with "fight-or-flight" stress responses, while parasympathetic has to do with relaxation responses. Autonomic nervous system imbalances have been linked with many diseases, allergic hyper-reactivity, and widespread effects influencing all parts of the body. Cranial osteopathy can be an extremely effective modality for treating arthritis, as well as many other disease conditions.

As you've read in this chapter, osteoarthritis is a complex problem with multiple contributing factors requiring a comprehensive holistic approach to effectively treat it. OMT is nearly always successful in allowing the patient greater mobility and a reduction in pain. This helps patients with arthritis to develop greater tolerance for exercise, which in turn will assist in controlling weight. It can be a valuable addition to the Arthritis Survival Program.

Naturopathic Medicine

Naturopathic physicians (N.D.'s) are specialists in natural medicine. They are trained at four-year naturopathic medical colleges and are educated in the conventional medical sciences. They treat both acute and chronic disease, and their treatments are drawn from clinical nutrition, herbal or botanical medicine, homeopathy, traditional Chinese medicine, physical medicine, exercise therapy, counseling, acupuncture, and hydrotherapy. Some naturopaths combine several or all of these therapies, whereas others specialize in one specific area. Dr. Todd Nelson, a naturopathic physician who is the co-creator of the Arthritis Survival Program, has great expertise in nutritional medicine.

The basic principles of naturopathy are based on the concept that the body is a self-healing organism. The naturopathic physician enhances the body's own natural immune response through non-invasive measures and health promotion. Rather than treat the symptoms, naturopaths strive to uncover the underlying cause of patients' diseases, looking at physical, mental, and emotional factors. Health is seen not as the absence of symptoms but as the absence of the causes of symptoms.

Prevention and wellness are vital principles in naturopathy. These physicians are trained to know which patients they can treat safely and which ones they need to refer to other health care practitioners. As teachers, naturopaths facilitate the growth of patients' responsibility for their own health and spark the enthusiasm and motivation patients need to make fundamental lifestyle changes. The origins of naturopathic philosophy extend as far back as Hippocrates, who set forth the principles "Do no harm" and "Let your food be your medicine, and your medicine be your food."

As a distinct American health care profession, naturopathic medicine is almost one hundred years old. Early in this century there were more than twenty naturopathic medical colleges. Today there are only four. In the 1940's and 1950's, with the advent of more technological medicine, the increased popularity of pharmaceutical drugs, and the belief that such drugs can eliminate all disease, naturopathy experienced a decline. During the past two decades, however, as more people have begun to seek alternatives to conventional medicine, it has seen a resurgence in popularity. N.D.'s are currently licensed in fourteen states.

Naturopathy seems to be making its greatest contributions to the healing arts in the fields of immunology, clinical nutrition, detoxification and botanical medicine. The diet, and much of the vitamin and herbal regimen for the treatment of arthritis and the strengthening of the immune system described in this chapter, come from naturopathic medicine.

Traditional Chinese Medicine

Traditional Chinese medicine is the primary health care system currently used by approximately 30 percent of the world's population. It is believed to be one of the oldest medical systems in existence, dating back almost five thousand years. The practice of acupuncture (a method of using fine needles to stimulate invisible lines of energy running beneath the surface of the skin) is the component of Chinese medicine most familiar to Americans, but the system also includes Chinese herbology, moxabustion (the burning of an herb at acupuncture points), massage, diet, exercise, and meditation.

In ancient China, doctors were not paid if patients under their care became sick. The job of the physician was to keep patients healthy. Chinese medicine believes that a certain process happens before the body develops a problem or disease. A Chinese medicine practitioner (O.M.D., doctor of oriental medicine) looks for this process or pattern of disharmony. Through questioning, observation, and palpation, a practitioner can determine a person's current state of health and the problems that individual will be at highest risk for developing in the future. In this way Chinese medicine is an effective preventive therapy.

Traditional Chinese medicine is based on a history, philosophy, and sociology very different from those of the West. Over thousands of years it has developed a unique understanding of how the body works. Practitioners of Chinese medicine see disease as an imbalance between the body's nutritive substances, called yin, and the functional activity of the body, called yang. This imbalance causes a disruption of the flow of vital energy that circulates through pathways in the body known as meridians. This vital energy, called *qi* or *chi,* keeps the blood circulating, warms the body, and fights disease. The intimate connection between the organ systems of the body and the meridians enables the practice of acupuncture to intercede and rebalance the body's energy through stimulation of specific points along the meridians.

People who have used Chinese medicine for a particular physical symptom frequently experience improvement in seemingly unrelated problems. This occurs because the Chinese approach tends to restore the body to a greater degree of balance, thereby enhancing its capacity for self-healing. The entire person is treated, not just the symptom, and the relationship of body, mind, emotions, spirit, and environment are all taken into account.

The World Health Organization has published a list of over fifty diseases successfully treated with acupuncture. Included on the list are arthritis, sinusitis, asthma, the common cold, headaches (including migraine), constipation, diarrhea, sciatica, and lower back pain. Acupuncture has also been effective in the treatment of allergies, addictions, insomnia, stress, depression, infertility, and menstrual problems.

Chinese herbs are the most common element of Chinese medicine as it is currently practiced in China. The herbs are becoming more popular in the United States, but it is still much easier to find a licensed acupuncturist (L.Ac., C.A., R.Ac., Dipl.

Ac.) than an O.M.D. who is knowledgeable about Chinese herbs as well as acupuncture. Since 1995 there has been national board certification in Chinese herbal medicine, offering the degree Dipl. C.H. As more schools of traditional Chinese medicine are established in this country, these licensed practitioners will be much easier to find.

Pharmaceutical drugs are usually made by synthetically producing the active ingredient of an herb. Medicinal plants differ from the isolated active ingredients in synthetic drugs because they contain associate substances that balance the medicinal effects. Uncomfortable side effects are generally the result of the removal of these associate substances. Chinese herbs are capable of regenerating, vitalizing, and balancing the vital energy, tissue, and organs of the body without harmful side effects. They can be taken in pill or powder form or as raw herbs made into tea.

In Traditional Chinese Medicine, emphasis is placed on ensuring that a person's energy and blood flow is smooth and harmonious. In people with arthritis the flow of blood and energy (*qi*) has been disrupted, which can lead to bone degeneration, pain, and/or swelling. Additionally, in accordance with Chinese medical theory, the kidney system (channel/meridian) "governs" the bones. In diseases that affect the bones, specifically their formation and integrity, there is a weakness in the kidney system. As we age, the kidney energy naturally weakens, which can lead to bone degeneration and many types of arthritis. This also explains the high incidence of arthritis amongst the elderly and post-menopausal women.

There can be many associated factors affecting the development and progression of osteoarthritis. When seeking treatment from an acupuncturist/doctor of oriental medicine, these factors will be taken into consideration. The primary focus of treatment is to move and regulate the flow of energy (*qi*) and blood and support the kidney energy. Usually, within four to six treatments, there will be a significant reduction in pain and/or swelling.

Simple self-care treatments for arthritis are available by using a few topical products that usually can be purchased at a health food store. They include: Zheng Gu Shul (linament), Po Sum On (massage medium), and Chinese herbal plasters.

Homeopathic Medicine

Homeopathy is a form of treatment that gently nudges the body toward a healthier state. Its practice was begun in 1820 by Samuel Hahnemann, a German physician, who believed that whatever caused disease would also cure it. The Latin phrase *similia similibus curantur* ("Like shall be cured by like") is the cornerstone of homeopathic medicine. According to Hahnemann, the proper remedy for an illness that exhibits any set of symptoms in a sick person is that substance that would produce the same set of symptoms in a healthy person.

This "law of similars" was not original with Hahnemann. The idea had been advanced by philosophers and physicians for thousands of years, and Hahnemann acknowledged his debt to Hippocrates, in whose writings the principle of "Like cures like" appears. Hahnemann, however, was the first to build a consistent system based on this principle.

Homeopathy flourished in the 1800's and hasn't changed much since then. The Hahnemann School of Medicine in Philadelphia was originally a school of homeopathic medicine. The advent of rigorous scientific medicine in the United States during this century almost completely eliminated homeopathy. Today this healing discipline is once again on the rise all over the world, including this country. The National Center for Homeopathic Medicine in Washington, D.C., estimates that there are somewhere between one and two thousand practitioners in the United States and that about three hundred of them are M.D.'s or D.O.'s. Homeopathy has fared much better in other parts of the world. One third of all French physicians practice it. In Britain, members of the royal family have been cared for by homeopathic physicians since the reign of Queen Victoria. Homeopathy is taught and used in hospitals and physicians' offices in Scotland, Germany, Austria, Switzerland, India, Mexico, Chile, Brazil, and Argentina.

Homeopathy uses infinitesimal or microdoses of natural materials—that is, mineral, plant, or animal. Some standard homeopathic solutions may be as weak as one part in a hundred thousand. These mixtures must be shaken vigorously (succussed) in a carefully prescribed manner in order to be activated. Only tiny amounts of a substance are used, but homeopaths believe that the treatment works because even if the substance were reduced to a single molecule, or lost altogether, its "pattern" would remain in the liquid and could produce an effect.

Scientific support for this theory was contained in a 1988 issue of the prestigious British journal *Nature*. The publication described a study from a French laboratory headed by a well-known medical research scientist in the fields of allergy and immunology. The research team demonstrated that a solution that had contained a human antibody, yet was so diluted that not a molecule of it was left, had produced a response in human blood cells. Science cannot explain precisely how this could happen, but the reasons why many pharmaceutical drugs, including aspirin, are effective are also still largely a mystery.

Homeopathic medicines are not required to meet the safe and effective standards of the Food and Drug Administration. They are sold by mail, in drugstores, and in health food stores. Most are nonprescription and can be legally advertised as remedies only for self-limiting conditions, such as colds. Prescription homeopathic substances can be dispensed only by someone licensed to prescribe drugs.

Many patients who seek the care of a homeopathic practitioner have a chronic condition considered incurable by conventional medicine. Most licensed, certified, or well-trained practitioners will often spend two or more hours in an initial evaluation. From that first comprehensive session they will prescribe one or more homeopathic remedies that specifically address your unique personality and dis-ease condition. There is no substitute for this type of thorough evaluation, and homeopathic remedies are best prescribed by a homeopathic practitioner. However, the following remedies may be helpful for providing relief from joint pain:

- **Rhus toxicodendron**—when the arthritis symptoms include pain and stiffness, and for aching joints that are worse in the morning and better from heat and continued movement.
- **Bryonia**—for swollen joints and pain that is aggravated by the slightest movement.
- **Arnica**—for a sore, bruised feeling in the joints, made worse by touch.
- **Rhododendron**—when pain is worse in stormy weather.

Ayurvedic Medicine (Ayurveda)

This branch of traditional Indian medicine is, along with traditional Chinese medicine, one of the oldest and most complete medical systems ever devised. Recognizing the integral relationship between body, mind, and spirit, Ayurvedic physicians view disease primarily as an imbalance in a person's life force (known as *prana*) and his or her predominant *dosha,* or basic metabolic condition. The three primary doshas are *pitta, vata,* and *kapha.* Restoring balance to the *doshas* and a person's pranic energy is the goal of Ayurveda. This is accomplished using diet, medicinal herbs, *pancha karma* (detoxification), *pranayama* (breathing exercises), and the most well-known components of Ayurveda in the West, meditation and yoga. For treating arthritis, Boswellia cream, camphor, and eucalyptus oil are used in addition to the above therapies. Oil massages of the affected joints, a therapeutic diet, along with Ayurvedic herbs, can also be beneficial for arthritis.

Chiropractic

Developed over one hundred years ago by David Daniel Palmer, the goal of chiropractic (Greek for "done by hand") is to maintain the health of the nervous system through the adjustment of bones and joints. Chiropractic theory holds that spinal misalignment (called subluxation) interferes with the flow of vital energy, or what Palmer described as the body's "innate intelligence." Since the nervous system's primary pathway is along the spine, when any part of the spine is subluxated, nerve impulses can be impeded and eventually result in dis-ease in the body's various organs. Chiropractors (or D.C.'s) restore spinal alignment with a variety of adjustment and manipulation techniques and comprise a large portion of the alternative practitioners in the United States. Many chiropractors also use kinesiology (muscle testing) and provide nutritional counseling in their practices. Chiropractic can be very helpful in treating arthritis (see study on page 59), especially when pain has resulted from misaligned or subluxated vertebra.

Energy Medicine

This includes a wide range of subtle bioenergetic techniques and the use of both conventional and experimental microcurrent and magnetic energy devices. Energy medicine may well become one of the most important aspects of holistic medicine in the twenty-first century, due to its use in diagnosing and treating disease in the human bioenergy field, often before it manifests physically in the body. Bioenergetic therapies within the field of energy medicine include Therapeutic Touch, healing touch, Reiki, and *jin shin jyutsu*. Distance healing, prayer, and meditation are other aspects of energy medicine, as are light, color, sound, and music therapies. Magnetic therapy, tai chi, and *qigong*, and microcurrent therapies (using devices such as the Acuscope and cranial electrical stimulation tools) also fall under the heading of energy medicine. Most of these therapies have the potential to improve the flow of blood and life force energy (*qi, prana*, or bioenergy) to the arthritic joint. In the hands of a skilled practitioner nearly all of these therapies can alleviate arthritis. I personally have had a positive experience in treating joint pain with healing touch and Reiki.

Bodywork and Body Movement

The various therapies within the category of bodywork and body movement all focus on restoring structural alignment and posture, creating unrestricted movement, and relieving physical tension and stress. *Rolfing*, more properly known as Structural

Integration, was developed by Ida Rolf, Ph.D. (1896–1979). Her doctorate in biochemistry and physiology, combined with years of study of other bodywork techniques, led her to conclude that all physiological function is an expression of structure. Her belief led her to develop her own system of bodywork as a way to cure her spinal arthritis. She realized that the physiologic conditions that contributed to causing arthritis could be resolved by stretching fascial tissues.

In Rolf's view, a body that is poorly aligned must struggle to maintain balance in the face of gravitational pull. As it does so, the body tends to compensate for areas of imbalance or misalignment in one area through adaptive changes in other areas. Over time, according to Rolfers (as practitioners of Rolfing are called), such compensation leads to an overall weakening of the body's entire structure, resulting in compromised body function. The aim of Rolfing is to restore the body to proper alignment so that all of its sections—head, neck, shoulders, torso, hips, legs, ankles, and feet—correspond and interact correctly with gravity. Rolf maintained that when the body's alignment is restored, all systems of the body are able to operate more efficiently, thereby improving total well-being.

Depending upon the degree of misalignment, Rolfing can take several months or even years to fully restore optimal positioning and function. During a Rolfing session, deep pressure is applied to the fascia, layers of connective tissue that hold and support the body's muscles and bones, and cover muscle fibers and internal organs. Due to injury and chronic stress, the fascia can shorten or become overly thick as a result of the body's adaptive coping strategies. Poor posture, disease, and emotional trauma can also contort the fascia. As a consequence, rigidity or over-solidity can occur, leading to habitual body distortion, spinal misalignment, limited range of motion, and repressed emotions. Rolfers seek to reestablish proper alignment and improve mobility by loosening and manipulating the fascia, using their fingers, thumbs, and sometimes elbows.

Rolfing, like most forms of bodywork, does not focus on

treating specific symptoms. Rather, emphasis is placed on bringing the body back into alignment with gravity by restoring the fascia to its natural state of elasticity. Although Rolfers make no claims of being able to treat specific disease conditions, Rolfing has been quite helpful in alleviating conditions of chronic pain and muscular tension, including lower back pain, and in improving posture. After curing her arthritis, Ida Rolf commented that "Many diagnoses of 'arthritis' reflect nothing more serious than a shortened or displaced muscle or ligament resulting from a recent or not-so-recent traumatic episode." I have personally had many Rolfing sessions with Jaison Kayn, a student of Ida Rolf, and found them to be one the most powerful holistic therapies (i.e., benefiting body, mind, and spirit) I've ever experienced.

Caution: Due to its deep manipulation of tissues, Rolfing is not advised for anyone suffering from acute pain or diseases due to underlying bone weakness, such as osteoporosis or fracture. Patients suffering from organic or inflammatory conditions, such as cancer or rheumatoid arthritis, or from acute skin inflammation, should also forgo Rolfing treatment.

Hellerwork was developed by Joseph Heller, one of Ida Rolf's early students and the first president of the Rolf Institute. Besides employing deep-touch techniques similar to those used by Rolfers to structurally realign the body, Hellerwork practitioners also seek to impart to their clients a greater awareness of the relationship between mind and body. To this end they utilize movement reeducation techniques and verbal dialog to address the complex interrelationship between the body's mechanical, psychological, and energetic functioning. Hellerwork usually consists of eleven sessions, each of which lasts for ninety minutes and makes use of a thematic approach that is geared toward providing clients with a structure for organizing the emotional aspects of the work. In the first session, for example, treatment is focused on resolving tension and unconscious holding patterns in the chest in order to bring about fuller, more natural breathing. During this session a Hellerwork practitioner will typically also engage clients in a dialog meant to call attention to his or her attitudes and emotions that may be affecting the breathing process. Instruction in proper movement is also provided in order to train clients in more efficient ways of using their body's energy and minimizing mechanical stress. Clients learn how to stand, sit, walk, run, and lift objects in a manner that is best suited to their own physiology. Videotaping of a client's movements may also be used to provide feedback and a clearer understanding of how movement patterns may need to be corrected. This form of bodywork can also be helpful in treating arthritis.

The Feldenkrais Method was developed by physicist and engineer Moshe Feldenkrais after he suffered a serious knee injury. Rather than undergo surgery, Feldenkrais devoted himself to the study of the nervous system and human behavior. His research, along with his knowledge of physiology, anatomy, psychology, neurology, and the martial arts, led him to conclude that a person's self-image is crucial to how he or she thinks and functions in the world. In Feldenkrais's view, the human organism is a complex interrelated system of function and intelligence in which all movement reflects the condition of the nervous system as well as being the basis of self-awareness.

Central to the philosophy of the Feldenkrais Method is the belief that the central nervous system can be retrained, resulting in improved patterns of behavior and movement. Feldenkrais also emphasized the importance of proper breathing, viewing the breath as an essential aspect of movement. In order to help his students overcome lifetimes of habitual limiting movement and breathing patterns, Feldenkrais developed two teaching methods, *Functional Integration* and *Awareness Through Movement*.

Functional Integration is taught individually in hour-long sessions tailored to the specific needs of each client. Using gentle manipulation and movement exercises, practitioners guide clients through new, easier, and more efficient ways of moving. No attempt is made to alter the client's body structure. Instead, practitioners use touch to help clients discover their own most appropriate movement style.

Awareness Through Movement classes are taught in a group setting. Classes average forty-five minutes to an hour in length, during which time students are guided through a series of directed movements. By paying attention to each exercise, students acquire a greater awareness of how they move and of any unnecessary tension their movements may have. The exercises are gentle and often subtle, such as lifting one foot slightly off the floor. They may be performed while sitting or lying on the floor, standing, or while seated, and can be accompanied by verbal cues or imagery designed to facilitate a deeper awareness of how each student moves. All exercises are performed slowly, without straining. There are Feldenkrais practitioners and classes available in most cities.

The Trager Approach, or *Trager Work,* was developed by U.S. physician Milton Trager, M.D., a specialist in neuromuscular conditions and a former boxer, acrobat, and dancer. Trager theorized that pain and other health conditions can be permanently resolved by bypassing the conscious mind to access the unconscious mind directly. Although different from the Feldenkrais Method, the goals of the Trager Approach are largely the same: releasing chronic and habitual tension in the body by helping clients recognize and interrupt limiting or inefficient movement patterns and correcting poor posture. One result of the attainment of these goals is less restricted movement and blood flow to painful or arthritic joints.

The Trager Approach is distinguished by the playful quality of its work, which achieves its goals through gentle, rhythmic touch and movement exercises. As the work is performed, the client lies passively on a massage table or flat surface, letting the practitioner guide the movements from a meditative state known as "hook up," which enables him or her to more deeply perceive the client's flow of energy. Limbs are lightly cradled and moved about in order to retrain the unconscious, via the nervous system, to move beyond old patterns of restriction and holding, into a state of greater flexibility and ease.

Caution: The Trager Approach is safe for most people, but should be avoided in cases of broken bones, fever, blood clotting, problem pregnancies, and certain forms of cancer, where manipulation might contribute to the spread of the disease.

Summary

Obviously the entire physical health component of the Arthritis Survival Program is too comprehensive for anyone to be expected to follow every one of these recommendations. However, there are many people who have obtained significant relief from their arthritis by strictly adhering to just *one* of the components of the program—the diet, or glucosamine, or SAMe, or fish oil, or Boswellia, etc. Dr. Nelson and I suggest to patients: *Make a commitment to incorporate into your daily life as many of the above recommendations as you are comfortably able to do.* Take your time. The more gradual the process the more likely it is that you'll stay with it. Try adding one new thing each week.

If, after three months of consistently adhering (daily practice) to at least three of the above recommendations, you have not yet experienced any change in your symptoms, we would continue with the initial dietary and supplement recommendations and also consider one of the *professional care therapies.* We would also suggest you begin to add the mental/emotional and spiritual/ social aspects (chapters 5 and 6) of the Arthritis Survival Program to the holistic approach for treating your arthritis. Remember, holistic medicine looks at every physical dis-ease as the body's reflection of an imbalance or disharmony in the whole person. *Healing* your degenerative joint disease entails more than simply modifying your diet or taking an herb or supplement. It may be helpful for you to work with a *holistic physician.* Please refer to the Resource Guide on page 195 to find one.

If you have followed the Arthritis Survival Program closely for at least three months, you will most likely have noticed a significant improvement. If so, you can begin to gradually relax the diet and the highest dosages of the supplements. There is no hard-and-fast rule for what the new dosages should be. Every individual is somewhat different, and you'll have to find the appropriate level for you. If your symptoms begin to recur, then increase to previous dosages. You can also gradually increase your level of exercise. To maintain and enhance your improvement, you can also start incorporating the following *physical and environmental health recommendations for optimal well-being,* in addition to the suggestions for "Healing the Mind" and "Healing the Spirit" in the next two chapters. Your commitment to these other two components of the Arthritis Survival Program is essential for *preventing recurrences* and possibly *curing your arthritis.*

PHYSICAL AND ENVIRONMENTAL HEALTH RECOMMENDATIONS FOR OPTIMAL WELL-BEING

Diet

There is no one universal diet that ideally suits every individual. Certain lab tests (including blood type), a comprehensive nutritional history, and personal experimentation (trial and error), along with the guidance of a holistic physician, can assist you in determining the diet best suited to your unique requirements. The following guidelines, however, are self-care approaches to establishing a diet from which almost anyone can derive significant health benefits.

The importance of a healthy diet in relationship to health has been emphasized for centuries in both the East and the West. While proper diet alone may not be enough to entirely reverse certain types of disease (this is true of arthritis), most chronic medical conditions can be significantly improved by a diet of nutrient-rich foods and adequate intake of purified water. Unfortunately, our society, with its over-reliance on fast foods and snacks, affords great temptation to stray from healthy eating habits. And even when we do resolve to change our diet for the better, many of us wind up confused about what foods to actually eat and how they should be prepared, due in great part to the steady introduction of best-selling books touting the "latest and greatest" cure-all diet. While such books may be well intentioned, not all of them contain scientifically supported recommendations, and those that do often contradict equally researched published information that made the best-seller list the year before. As a result, a number of polls now indicate that growing numbers of Americans are literally "fed up" with the amount of dietary and nutritional information that is becoming increasingly prevalent in our society.

A good dose of common sense can go a long way toward alleviating this confusion. There is a great deal of truth to the old adage "You are what you eat." The foods you consume become the fuel your body uses to carry out its countless functions. Therefore, it makes good sense to eat those foods that are the best "fuel sources." This means foods that are rich in vitamins, minerals, enzymes, essential fatty and amino acids, and other necessary nutrients, and are free of preservatives, pesticides, and other substances that deplete the body's energy and can damage your vital organs. Dr. Todd Nelson's recommended diet, the *New Life Eating Plan* (NLEP), is the one I follow and suggest to my patients. Earlier in this chapter we outlined Phase I of the NLEP for the initial stages of rebalancing body chemistry to help restore optimal function and heal your arthritic joint(s). Phase I serves as the basis of healthy eating for those who are experiencing chronic illness. Phase II, at the end of this section (page 97), allows for some dietary expansion and food rotation.

Rethinking the American Way of Eating

In January 1992 the U.S. Department of Agriculture (USDA) unveiled its recommended dietary pyramid as a guideline for meeting these nutritional needs (see Figure 3). At the base of this pyramid are whole grains, such as brown rice, bulgur, wheat (breads and pasta), oats, barley, millet, and cereals, with a recommended six to eleven servings from this food group per day.

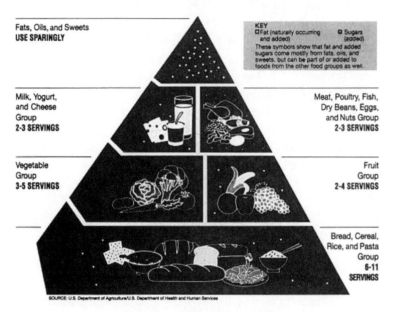

Food Guide Pyramid

A Guide to Daily Food Choices

Fats, Oils, and Sweets
USE SPARINGLY

KEY
□ Fat (naturally occurring ▢ Sugars
and added) (added)
These symbols show that fat and added
sugars come mostly from fats, oils, and
sweets, but can be part of or added to
foods from the other food groups as well.

Milk, Yogurt,
and Cheese
Group
2-3 SERVINGS

Meat, Poultry, Fish,
Dry Beans, Eggs,
and Nuts Group
2-3 SERVINGS

Vegetable
Group
3-5 SERVINGS

Fruit
Group
2-4 SERVINGS

Bread, Cereal,
Rice, and Pasta
Group
**6-11
SERVINGS**

SOURCE: U.S. Department of Agriculture/U.S. Department of Health and Human Services

FIGURE 3.   *Food Guide Pyramid*

The next section of the pyramid is divided into the categories of
fruits and vegetables, with a recommended two to four servings
of the former and three to five servings of the latter. Moving
upward, we find a recommended two to three servings each of
dairy products (milk, yogurt, and cheese) and the meats, poultry, fish, eggs, dry beans, and nut group. Fats, oils, and sweets are
at the top and should be used sparingly.

While the USDA food pyramid can be a useful place to start,
a number of recent studies now indicate that our daily need for
carbohydrates from whole grains may not be as vital as our need
for fresh fruits and vegetables. A good deal of this research has
been popularized by Dr. Barry Sears, Ph.D., in his book *The*

Zone Diet. He and other researchers have found that there are a variety harmful effects resulting from excessive intake of carbohydrates, especially those that have a high *glycemic index* (they break down quickly and release glucose into the blood at a rapid rate). (See pages 81–83.) These ill effects include:

- **Overstimulation of insulin production,** which can lead to excess storage of fat in the body, hypoglycemia, increased inflammation, cardiac risk, and diabetes
- **Diminished physical and mental capacity**
- **Fluctuating energy levels and mood swings**
- **Predisposition to other chronic diseases,** including arthritis, heart disease, and skin disorders.

As a result, practitioners of holistic medicine now place more emphasis on the fruit and vegetable groups, recommending more servings of these two food groups over whole grains, breads, pasta, and cereal. Flour-based food—bread, pasta, and bagels—have a very high glycemic index. Whole grains, beans, and legumes, and most starchy vegetables, except potatoes, have a low glycemic index and are emphasized in the NLEP.

It is also recommended that milk—other than 1 percent or skim—be eliminated, and that your daily intake of butter, margarine, and cheese be reduced.

Beyond the USDA Food Pyramid

Dr. Nelson developed the NLEP after realizing that all of his chronically ill patients were making at least six critical dietary mistakes. These six were part of a list that he identified as the fifteen most common mistakes in the American diet that undermine health. They are:

(1) Excess saturated fat, trans fats, cooked fats, and insufficient essential fatty acids (EFAs)
(2) Excess sweets
(3) Excess refined carbohydrates and insufficient complex carbohydrates

TABLE 4.3

Glycemic Index

Carbohydrates act like a powerful drug elevating insulin in the body. This in turn can increase fat deposits, LDL cholesterol (the unhealthy kind), and inflammation, while decreasing immunity. The amount of insulin the body produces is based on the amount of carbohydrates that actually enters the bloodstream as the simple sugar glucose. This is why you can consume a large amount of the 3-percent or 6-percent vegetables and fruits (refer to Table 4.4, Carbohydrate Classifications of Fruits and Vegetables, p. 83) in comparison to the amount of grains, starches, breads, or pastas at any given meal.

Example: 1½ cups of broccoli, or any other 3-percent vegetable = ¼ cup pasta.

This is why it is best to focus on the low-density carbohydrates (3 percent and 6 percent). Not only can you eat more, but there are many other benefits, including high water content, high fiber content, vitamins, minerals and enzymes.

People are genetically designed to eat primarily fruits and vegetables as their major source of carbohydrates.

All carbohydrates, simple or complex, have to be broken down into simple sugars before being absorbed by the body and entering the bloodstream. The only simple sugar that can actually enter the bloodstream is glucose. The faster glucose enters the bloodstream, the more insulin you make. This is important for you to know when you are making your choice of carbohydrates. *The higher the glycemic index of carbohydrates, the faster it enters the bloodstream as sugar.*

Low Glycemic (Examples: 3-percent and 6-percent fruits and vegetables)
Fructose has to be converted into glucose via the liver, so fruits are a lower glycemic index than grains and starches.

High Glycemic (Examples: bagel, pasta, cooked starches)
Cornflakes are pure glucose linked by chemical bonds. These bonds are easily broken in the stomach and glucose rushes into the bloodstream. Table sugar is one half glucose and one half fructose, so it actually enters the bloodstream slower than a bagel.

There are other factors involved that have an effect on how fast the carbohydrates are broken down into simple sugar. Fat and soluble fibers slow the entry of glucose. Soluble fiber is an important distinction. There are two types of fiber, soluble (pectin, apples) and insoluble (cellulose and bran cereal). And because fat slows down the entry of glucose into the bloodstream, the sugar in ice cream actually is absorbed more slowly than that of a bagel. High fiber in low glycemic foods is the slowest to release sugars.

The more the carbohydrates are cooked, the higher the glycemic index will be. This is because the cell structure is broken down by cooking and processing. The glycemic index is dramatically increased in instant foods made from rice and potatoes. Therefore all bread has a high glycemic index.

Highest Glycemic Index Foods (Examples: puffed cereal and puffed rice cakes)

The body needs a constant intake of carbohydrates for optimal brain function. Too much carbohydrate and the body increases insulin secretion to drive down blood sugar. Too little and the brain will not function efficiently. High glycemic food should always be avoided with candida overgrowth.

Remember, protein stimulates glucagon, which reduces insulin secretion, while fat and fiber slow down the rate of entry of any carbohydrate.

(4) Excess alcohol

(5) Excess caffeine

(6) Excess salt

(7) Excess consumption of overly cooked food

(8) Excess processed and devitalized food

(9) Excess "high stress" protein sources and insufficient "low stress" protein sources

(10) Excess consumption of food-borne toxins (preservatives, mold, bacteria, additives, artificial sweeteners, colorings, flavoring, hydrogenated fats, heavy metals)

(11) Insufficient high quality, fresh organic produce—both fruits and vegetables

(12) Insufficient pure water

TABLE 4.4

Carbohydrate Classifications of Fruits and Vegetables

(According to Carbohydrate Content)

VEGETABLES

3%	6%	15%	20+%
asparagus	beans, string	artichoke	beans, dried
bean sprouts	beets	carrot	beans, lima
beet greens	brussels sprouts	oyster plant	corn
broccoli	chives	parsnip	potato, sweet
cabbage	collard greens	peas, green	potato, white
cauliflower	dandelion greens	squash	yam
celery	eggplant		
chard, swiss	kale		
cucumber	kohlrabi		
endive	leek		
lettuce	okra		
mustard greens	onion		
radish	parsley		
spinach	pepper, red		
watercress	pimento		
	pumpkin		
	rutabagas		
	turnip		

FRUITS

3%	6%	15%	20+%
cantaloupe	apricot (fresh only)	apple	banana
melons	blackberries	blueberries	figs
rhubarb	cranberries	cherries	prunes
strawberries	grapefruit	grapes	or any dried
tomato	guava	kumquats	fruit
watermelon	kiwi	loganberries	
	lemon	mango	
	lime	mulberries	
	melons	pear	
	orange	pineapple (fresh)	
	papaya	pomegranate	
	peach		
	plum		
	raspberries		
	tangerine		

(13) Insufficient balanced fiber intake
(14) Poor food combinations
(15) Stressful eating environment and insufficient chewing.

Consistently making poor choices in these fifteen areas over the course of a lifetime will usually result in poor health. This occurs from the cumulative effect of increased chemical toxicity, free radical damage, nutrient depletion, and dysbiosis resulting in immune, endocrine, neurologic, rheumatologic, and cardiac dysfunction.

Dr. Nelson has concluded that the goal of any dietary program for preventing and treating a chronic illness should be targeted at correcting these common mistakes and establishing a regenerative way of eating for life. This is the primary purpose of the New Life Eating Plan. As you begin to adopt these principles you'll soon realize that this diet is an essential component of the daily practice of loving and nurturing yourself.

Let's now explore some of the specific steps you can take in committing to the NLEP or a comparably healthy diet. Out of the fifteen most common mistakes, we will emphasize changing the first six on the list above. These are perhaps the most important mistakes that we commonly make, which we refer to as "The Sickening Six."

"The Sickening Six"

There are six substances in the American diet which should be substantially eliminated—unhealthy fats, sugar, refined carbohydrates, alcohol, caffeine, and salt. These "sickening six" can lead to a variety of disease conditions. While it is all right to enjoy these substances in moderation, keeping their intake to a minimum can pay big health dividends. Here are a number of reasons why:

(1) Unhealthy Fats

The regular intake of good fats, called essential fatty acids (EFAs), is essential to our health. (Refer to page 50.) Unfortunately, most of us are getting too much unhealthy fat in our diets. Primary sources of these harmful fats include red meats, milk, and other dairy products, and the hydrogenated trans fats found in margarine, cooking fats, and many brands of peanut butter. These fats are also found in many packaged foods, including most commercial cereals, which also tend to be loaded with sugar.

Unhealthy fats lead to arteriosclerosis, the buildup of plaque on the inner lining of the arteries, where over time they obstruct the flow of blood and the transport of oxygen and nutrients to the body's internal organs. This obstruction, in turn, can lead to heart attacks, angina, stroke, kidney failure, and pre-gangrene in the legs.

The excessive intake of unhealthy fats is also associated with certain cancers. Among them are cancer of the breast, colon, rectum, prostate, ovaries, and uterus. This is particularly true of the saturated fats derived from meat products.

Obesity, which is increasing to epidemic proportions in this country, is also directly related to excessive fat (and sugar) intake. Obesity is a serious disease condition by itself, but if prolonged, it can contribute to many other forms of illness, including adult-onset diabetes.

Becoming aware of your fat intake and minimizing the amount of harmful fats you consume is an important step toward optimal health.

(2) Sugar

The use of sugar in your diet can pose many harmful health risks; yet, the average American consumes 150 pounds each year. This is the equivalent of over forty teaspoons of sugar every day. The following are only a few of sugar's health-depleting effects:

- Sugar has been shown to be a risk factor for heart disease, diabetes, hypoglycemia, and syndrome X, *and may be more harmful than fat.*
- Sugar weakens the immune system, increasing susceptibility to infection and allergy and exacerbating all other diseases caused by diminished immune function.

- Sugar stimulates excessive insulin production, thereby causing more fat to be stored in the body; lowers HDL cholesterol levels (the healthy cholesterol); increases the production of harmful triglycerides; and increases the risk of arteriosclerosis (hardening of the arteries).
- Sugar contributes to diminished mental capacity and can cause feelings of anxiety, depression, and rage. It has also been implicated in certain cases of attention deficit disorder (ADD).
- High sugar intake is associated with certain cancers, including cancer of the gall bladder and colon. Recently, sugar has also been implicated as a causative factor in cases of breast cancer.
- Excessive sugar in the diet is a primary contributor to candidiasis (intestinal yeast overgrowth), which can lead to a host of health problems, including gastrointestinal disorders, asthma, bronchitis, sinusitis, allergies, and chronic fatigue.

If you still feel a need to satisfy your sweet tooth, substitute modest amounts of pure honey or maple syrup to decrease the risk of these adverse effects.

(3) Refined Carbohydrates

Refined, or simple, carbohydrates, such as those found in white breads, and pastas made from white flour, are another group of health-threatening agents. When eaten to excess, these types of foods overstimulate insulin production and produce the same excessive fat storage in the body that results from eating too much sugar. This can lead to the onset of diabetes and obesity. The rise in obesity among American children is due in part to a diet heavy in sugars and refined carbohydrates, and lacking in nutritious alternatives, notably fruits and vegetables.

Several recent studies have shown that certain carbohydrates previously promoted as being "whole" sources of starch are very rapidly digested and absorbed. As a result, they elevate blood sugar fully as much as sugar itself, contributing to all of the problems cited above in (2) Sugar. Most carbohydrates have been carefully analyzed and assigned a *glycemic index rating.* (For a rating of fruits and vegetables, refer to page 83.) A high glycemic index indicates that a food acts much like sugar in the body, while food sources with a low glycemic index are much slower to be assimilated and therefore offer much better nutritional value. High gylcemic index foods include corn flakes, puffed rice, instant and mashed potatoes, white bread, maltose, and, of course, sugar itself. Foods with a low glycemic index include whole grain cereals (oats, brown rice, amaranth, kamut, millet), legumes (beans, peas, soybeans), whole wheat pastas, pearled barley, bulgur wheat, sweet potatoes, root vegetables, yogurt, and fructose.

(4) Alcohol

Alcohol is another example of a substance that, when taken in moderation, may enhance health, but when consumed in excess can cause a variety of serious problems. A growing body of research now indicates that one or two beers or a glass of wine per day can be beneficial to health as a way to relieve stress and improve digestion. In fact, studies have shown that complete abstainers from alcohol have a slightly shorter life expectancy than those who drink in moderate amounts. Unfortunately, for many men especially, alcohol and moderation usually "don't mix."

Although most people drink in order to feel better, evidence indicates that alcohol can significantly contribute to feelings of depression, loneliness, restlessness, and boredom, according to studies conducted by the National Center for Health Statistics. In addition, very moody people are also three times as likely to be heavy drinkers (three or more drinks per day).

Aside from the social stigma surrounding excessive alcohol consumption, too much alcohol can also contribute to obesity; increased blood pressure; diabetes; colon, stomach, breast, mouth, esophagus, laryngeal, and pancreatic cancers; gastrointestinal disorders; impaired liver function; candidiasis; impaired mental functioning; and behavioral and emotional dysfunctions. If you are having difficulty in bringing your alcohol consumption under control, seek the help of a professional counselor.

(5) Caffeine

Caffeine is a drug to which more than half of all Americans are addicted. On average we drink at least two and a half cups of coffee a day, or 425 milligrams of caffeine. Because caffeine acts as a stimulant, we consume it in order to have more energy. But the quick-fix boost it provides usually only lasts for a few hours, leaving us with greater fatigue and irritability once its effects wear off. Typically, when this happens, we reach for another cup of coffee to keep us going. The result is a roller coaster of ups and downs which, over time, can result in a number of health hazards.

While caffeine in moderation (200 milligrams or less per day) is relatively safe, the regular consumption of greater amounts can result in elevated blood pressure; increased risk of cancer, heart disease, and osteoporosis; poor sleep patterns; anxiety and irritability; dizziness; impaired circulation; urinary frequency; and gastrointestinal disorders. I previously mentioned that drinking four cups of coffee per day can double the risk for developing arthritis. Caffeine also causes loss of calcium from muscle cells and can interfere with the blood clotting process by decreasing platelet stickiness.

Taken in moderation, however, caffeine has been shown to enhance mental functioning and improve both alertness and mood, suggesting that 200 milligrams or less of caffeine per day may be safely tolerated by most individuals. Depending upon whether you're drinking instant, percolated, or drip coffee, 200 milligrams is the equivalent of between one and two cups.

If you consider yourself addicted to caffeine, the best way to break your habit is to reduce your intake *very gradually,* over a period of a few weeks or even months. Start by substituting non-caffeinated drinks such as herbal tea or a roasted-grain beverage in place of one of your normal cups of coffee per day. Over time, cut back further while increasing the number of substitute beverages, and beware of possible withdrawal symptoms such as headache, nervousness, and irritability. Typically, these will pass within a day or two. Also avoid other caffeine sources, such as soft drinks (particularly colas), cocoa, chocolate, and nonherbal teas.

If you still choose to drink coffee, the least harmful choice is Swiss water-processed organic decaf.

(6) Salt

Salt is another ingredient that is far too prevalent in many diets, and it poses particular dangers for certain people who suffer from high blood pressure. Many of us have been conditioned since childhood to crave salt, but its overuse draws water into the bloodstream. This, in turn, increases blood volume, causing higher blood pressure levels. Too much salt also upsets the body's sodium-potassium balance, thereby interfering with the lymphatic system's ability to draw wastes away from the cells.

Although some salt can be used in cooking, a good rule of thumb is to avoid adding salt to your food once it is served.

Beginning the NLEP

As a starting point in changing your diet, reduce your intake of red meat, and when you do eat it, choose only the leanest cuts. In its place, have two to three servings per day of either fish, poultry, beans, or nuts. Also avoid all cooking fats and oils derived from animal products and those from vegetable sources that are hydrogenated and found in most margarines, many brands of peanut butter, and hydrogenated cooking fats. Instead, use vegetable oils, such as olive and canola. Flaxseed oil, a particularly rich source of vital omega-3 essential fatty acids, can also be used for healthy dressings (but not for cooking). The best fats are from whole vegetables and grains that are unprocessed, polyunsaturated, and non-oxidized.

Also pay attention to the various food additives that are commonly found in the typical American diet. These include all chemical preservatives, such as BHA, BHT, sodium nitrate, and sulfites; artificial coloring agents; and artificial sweeteners, such as saccharin, aspartame (NutraSweet), and cyclamates. These additives have the potential to be enormous health risks. To avoid their use, stay away from processed or canned foods and get in the habit of reading labels whenever you go shopping. If you can't pronounce the ingredient, then don't eat it.

Finally, if you aren't already in the habit of doing so, consider selecting fruits and vegetables that are grown organically, and meats and poultry derived from animals that are raised free-range and are chemical-free. In the former case, you will be eating foods that are richer in nutrients and free of pesticides, artificial fertilizers, preservatives and other additives. Free-range meats and poultry are the end products of animals that are not subject to irradiation or injections of growth hormones and antibiotics commonly found in meats and poultry raised commercially.

What follow, by category, are listings of a variety of nutritious foods that can be added to your diet for their rich nutrient value.

Fruits and Vegetables

Fresh fruits and vegetables, organic when possible, should be a staple of your daily diet as a primary source of carbohydrate. Not only are they rich with nutrients, they also possess vital cleansing properties and high fiber content, which help rid the body of waste and toxins, creating greater levels of energy. Be sure to eat at least part of your daily servings of fruits and vegetables raw, since in this form you will be receiving the highest nutrient content. Lightly steaming vegetables is another healthy way to prepare them. Boiling or overcooking vegetables, on the other hand, can destroy the abundant vitamins, minerals, and enzymes in these foods.

Among the fruits and vegetables with the greatest nutritional value (especially vitamin C, carotenes, and antioxidant value) are: blueberries, cherries, red grapes, plums, cantaloupe, strawberries, apples, guavas, red chili peppers, red and green sweet peppers, kale, parsley, greens (mustard, collard, and turnip), broccoli, cauliflower, Brussels sprouts, carrots, yams, spinach, mangoes, winter squash, romaine lettuce, asparagus, tomatoes, onions, garlic, peaches, papayas, bananas, grapefruit, watermelon, and sprouts.

Note: Although they are extremely rich sources of vitamins, minerals, and fiber, fruits impede the digestion of other foods and are therefore best eaten away from meals as snacks: 10 or more minutes before or 2 hours after a meal.

Whole Grains and Complex Carboydrates

Whenever possible, whole grains, beans, and legumes should be a primary source of carbohydrates as they, too, provide many essential vitamins and minerals. Most grains also supply about 10 percent of excellent quality protein. Among the recommended whole grains are amaranth, millet, brown rice, basmati rice, quinoa, barley, rye, and oats. Use wheat sparingly on a rotation basis according to NLEP Phase II. Other sources of complex carbohydrates are starchy vegetables and legumes. Complex carbohydrates provide sustained boosts of energy and digest slowly, releasing their sugars into the bloodstream gradually. This gradual release of sugars helps to maintain insulin balance and contributes to the production of adenosine triphosphate (ATP) in the cells, thereby strengthening the immune system. Good sources of starchy vegetables include sweet potatoes, yams, acorn and butternut squash, and pumpkins. For legumes, choose black beans, garbanzo beans (chickpeas), lima beans, adzuki beans, navy beans, kidney beans, lentils, black-eyed peas, or split peas.

Proteins

Proteins are the nutrients your body uses to build cells, repair tissue, and produce the basic building blocks of DNA and RNA. Bones, hair, nails, muscle fibers, collagen, and other connective tissues are all composed of protein, and protein itself is second only to water in terms of the body's overall composition.

The main sources of protein for a healthy diet are fish, chicken and turkey (select cuts that are free-range and free of hormones and antibiotics), healthy eggs, soy products (soy milk, tofu, miso, and tempeh), sunflower seeds, almonds, cashews, peanuts, pine nuts, pecans, walnuts, and sesame seeds. Red meats and dairy products are not on this list due to their higher concentration of unhealthy fats, which can contribute to inflammation, and to a host of disease conditions, especially heart disease and hardening of the arteries. Low- or nonfat organic cultured dairy products such as yogurt or cottage cheese are well tolerated by many people.

Fats and Oils

Contrary to popular belief, all of us need some fats in our diet. Fats supply energy reserves which the body draws upon when not enough fats are present in the foods we eat. Fats also serve as a primary form of insulation and help to maintain normal body temperature. In addition, fats help to transport oxygen; absorb fat soluble vitamins (A, D, E, and K); nourish the skin, mucous membranes, and nerves; and serve as an anti-inflammatory. Healthy fat is utilized by the body in the form of essential fatty acids (EFAs).

Excessive fat intake, however, can contribute to a variety of illnesses, especially obesity and heart disease. Fat intake that is too low can also pose health risks. One of the keys to optimal health, then, is to make sure that you are getting an adequate supply of fats in your diet, and that they are "good" fats, not fats that are harmful. These good fats, in the form of oils, remain liquid at room temperature.

The best food sources of healthy fats are the whole foods from which the oils are derived. These include foods such as nuts and seeds, soybeans, olives, and avocados. Healthy fats in the form of oils include olive, canola, flaxseed (do not use for cooking), and sesame. Essential fatty acids are found in two groups, the omega-3's and the omega-6's. Good sources of omega-3 include cold water fish (salmon, sardines, tuna, sole), wild game, flaxseeds and flaxseed oil, canola oil, walnuts, pumpkin seeds, soybeans, fresh sea vegetables, and leafy greens. Good sources of omega-6 include vegetable oils, legumes, all nuts and seeds, and most grains, organ meats, lean meats, leafy greens, borage oil, evening primrose oil, and gooseberry and black-currant oils.

Fiber

Fiber is one of the most overlooked components of a healthy diet, with the average American diet supplying only one fourth to one third of the amount necessary for optimal health. High-fiber diets are associated with less coronary heart disease, lower cholesterol and triglyceride levels, lower blood pressure, lower incidence of cancer (especially of the colon and rectum), better control of diabetes, and lower incidences of diverticulitis, appendicitis, gall bladder disease, ulcerative colitis, and hernias. Lack of fiber is also the major cause of constipation and hemorrhoids.

Fiber includes the nondigestible substances in the foods that we eat. Good sources of fiber include fruits; the bran portion of whole grains, such as whole wheat, rolled oats, and brown rice; and raw and cooked green, yellow, and starchy vegetables, such as spinach, romaine lettuce, squash, carrots, beans, and lentils. The goal is 25 to 35 grams of fiber intake per day.

Water

Next to oxygen, water is our most essential nutrient, and drinking enough water to satisfy your body's needs may be the simplest, least expensive self-help measure you can adopt to maintain your good health.

Our adult bodies are 60 to 70 percent water (an infant's body is about 80 percent), and water is the medium through which every bodily function occurs. It is the basis of all body fluids, including blood, digestive juices, urine, lymph, and perspiration, which explains why, without water, we would die within a few days.

Water is vital to metabolism and digestion and helps prevent both constipation and diarrhea. It is also critical to healthy nerve-impulse conduction and brain function. Some of water's other vital functions in the body are:

- enhancing oxygen uptake into the bloodstream (The surface of the lungs must be moistened with water to facilitate oxygen intake and excretion of carbon dioxide.)
- maintaining a high urine volume, helping to prevent kidney stones and urinary tract infections
- regulating body temperature through perspiration
- maintaining and increasing the health of the skin

- maintaining adequate fluid for the lubrication of the joints and enhancing muscular function, particularly during and after exercise or other strenuous activity
- moistening the mucous membranes of the respiratory tract, which in turn increases resistance to infection and allows the sinuses to drain more easily.

Because water is so important to our health, all of us need to make a conscious effort to stay well hydrated, since most of us lose water faster than we replace it. For example, we lose one pint of water each day simply through exhalation. We also lose the same amount through perspiration, as well as three additional pints per day through urination and defecation. Exercise and heat exposure, especially in a dry climate, also increase water loss in the body. The percentage of body-water content also decreases with age. All told, on average, each of us loses two and a half quarts of water (80 ounces) per day under normal conditions. Therefore, it is essential that the same amount or more be replenished daily.

Unfortunately, most Americans don't come close to consuming that much water per day. As a result, many of us are chronically dehydrated. When we think of dehydration, we may envision a lost soul in the desert dying of thirst. However, most conditions of dehydration are not that dramatic, making dehydration all too often unsuspected and therefore undiagnosed. Meanwhile, its insidious effects can wreak havoc on our health by chronically impacting every one of our bodily functions. The results are:

- reduced blood volume, with less oxygen and nutrients provided to all muscles and organs
- reduced brain size and impaired neuromuscular coordination, concentration, and thinking
- excess body fat
- poor muscle tone and size
- impaired digestive function and constipation
- increased toxicity in the body

- joint and muscle pain
- water retention (edema), which can result in a state of being overweight and also impede weight loss
- hyperconcentration of blood with increased viscosity, leading to higher risk of heart attack.

Even though you may not be feeling thirsty, you may nonetheless be one of the millions of Americans who are chronically dehydrated. Observation of your urine is one simple way to determine if you are. If your urine is heavy, cloudy, and deep yellow, orange, or brown in tint, more than likely you are dehydrated. The urine of a properly hydrated body tends to be light and nearly clear in color, similar in appearance to unsweetened lemonade. As your water intake approaches your daily need for it, you will notice the appearance of your urine changing accordingly. (Remember that B vitamins will also turn urine a dark yellow.)

Because dehydration is so deceptive—it can occur without symptoms of thirst—in general, we need to drink more water than our thirst calls for. This does not mean coffee, soft drinks, or alcohol, all of which further contribute to dehydration. Even processed fruit juices and milk are not healthy substitutes for water because of the sugar and possible pesticides in the former, and hormones and antibiotics in the latter.

The exact amount of water a person needs depends on a number of individual factors, such as body weight, diet, metabolic rate, climate, level of physical activity, and stress factors. Some health professionals recommend that we all drink eight 8-ounce glasses of water a day. A more accurate rule of thumb is to drink half an ounce of water per pound of body weight if you are a healthy but sedentary adult, and to increase that amount to two thirds of an ounce per pound if you are an active exerciser. This means that a healthy, sedentary adult weighing 160 pounds should drink about ten 8-ounce glasses of water, while an active exerciser should drink thirteen to fourteen 8-ounce glasses. If your diet is particularly high in fresh fruits and vegetables, your daily water intake needs may be less, since these foods are 85 to 90 percent water content and can help restore lost fluids. Herbal teas, natural fruit juices (without sugar and diluted 50 percent with water), and soups that are sugarless and low in salt (the thinner the better) are also acceptable substitutes for drinking water.

Nearly as important as the amount of water you drink is the *quality* of your water. Simply put, if you aren't drinking filtered water, then your body is forced to become the filter. Still, it's impossible to generalize about whether you should drink tap, bottled, or filtered water. (Distilled water is not recommended for drinking because it lacks necessary minerals and can also leach them from your body.) In some communities, water purity is so high that it requires no treatment, while other water sources are contaminated with high concentrations of lead and radon, the two worst contaminants.

Another issue regarding our drinking water is chlorination. Since chlorine was first introduced into America's drinking water supply in 1908, it has eliminated epidemics of cholera, dysentery, and typhoid. Multiple studies, however, now suggest an association between chlorine and increased free-radical production, which can lead to a higher incidence of cancer. On the positive side, chlorine is effective in eliminating most microorganisms from drinking water. (One notable exception is the parasite *Cryptosporidium,* which is resistant to chlorine.)

Unless you live in one of the communities that supplies pure water, drinking tap water is not recommended, especially since the majority of health-related risks present in drinking water occur from contamination that is added *after* the water leaves the treatment and distribution plant. This includes pipes that run from municipal systems into your home, lead-soldered copper pipes, and fixtures that contain lead and may leach lead or other toxic metals (such as cadmium, mercury, and cobalt) into your tap water. Therefore, if you drink tap water, it would be a good idea to have the water from your tap tested, regardless of the claims from your local water utility. You can get started by calling your local health department for a referral for testing.

Because of the growing concerns regarding tap water, increasing numbers of Americans now choose bottled water for drinking and cooking purposes. Not only can this prove to be expensive, it also may not be as safe as you think. Regulations mandated for the bottled-water industry are similar to those followed by the public water treatment industry, and currently do not include required testing for *Cryptosporidium* and many other contaminants. Moreover, 25 percent of bottled water sold in this country comes from filtered municipal water that is then treated. For this reason, perhaps the healthiest choice regarding your drinking water is to invest in a water filter.

Since it is impossible to always know for certain whether what we drink or eat is completely safe, do the best you can. To get in the habit of drinking enough water, spread your intake throughout the day (drinking very little after dinner) and don't drink more than four 8-ounce glasses in any one-hour period. It's also best to drink between meals so as not to interfere with your body's digestive process. Make your water drinking convenient: Keep a container of water at hand, in your car or at your desk, and don't wait until you feel thirsty to start drinking.

The New Life Eating Plan, Phase II

Now that you have been on Phase I for three to six months, you are ready to expand your food choices. Hopefully you have been able to stick to Phase I very closely and are reaping the benefits of renewed vitality, less pain, greater joint mobility, better digestion, and an enthusiastic commitment to your self-care. At this point it is natural for you to desire more variety in your food choices. But be careful! Many people will experience great results from eating like this and then adopt the attitude "I've been doing well, so now I can go back to some of the old foods that I love." In fact, you may be tempted to go overboard in the opposite direction. The worst that can happen is that you will start feeling pain in your joints again. This is simply your body wisely reminding you to get back to a healthy diet. Let's now look at a safe, gradual way to expand your choices while continuing to minimize toxicity and allergic reactions, and maximize nutrient density.

At this point in your Arthritis Survival Program, try allowing the following list of foods back into your diet. Allow them only one at a time every four to six days so you can be more aware of symptoms and track any food reactions. Score your symptoms each day on the symptom chart. If your symptoms seem to increase within a 24- to 72-hour period, and you haven't made any other significant dietary changes, then you are probably reacting to that new food and should continue to avoid it. If you are unsure, keep that food out of your diet for seven days and re-test it.

Once you know you tolerate a food, allow it on a rotational basis, which means once every three to five days. For example, if you have a wheat product on Monday, wait until Thursday to have it again so your body has a chance to clear any reactions it may have to it. This also helps you to prevent developing a reaction to that specific food.

Foods to test rotating back into your diet

(These are foods to generally de-emphasize in the diet and are not required to be healthy. They should only be allowed back in if you enjoy them and you continue to feel well while eating them.)

- wheat
- corn
- bananas
- cheese
- cultured dairy: nonfat yogurt or cottage cheese
- red meat (Avoid pork products over the long term.)
- citrus fruit
- whole-grain rye crackers
- higher glycemic foods: flour-based foods such as whole grain pasta, bread, pancakes, muffins, and starchier fruits and vegetables (Use *very* sparingly.)
- small amounts of sweetener: Stevia is best, or honey, maple syrup, or brown rice syrup.

Remember: It's what you do most of the time—day in and day out—with your diet that counts. Maintain a lot of variety, so you won't get bored. Do the best you can. Your joints will let you know if you need to do better.

Nutritional Supplements

"I believe that you can, by taking some simple and inexpensive measures, extend your life and your years of well-being. My most important recommendation is that you take vitamins every day to optimum amounts, to supplement the vitamins you receive in your food."

LINUS PAULING, PH.D., two-time Nobel Prize laureate,

who lived a full and productive 93 years by following his own advice

Following the dietary recommendations outlined above is a vital first step in creating optimal health for yourself and your loved ones. Sadly, however, a healthy diet alone, even one that is rich with pure, organically grown foods, is no longer enough to ensure total physical well-being. Due to our unhealthy environment (see below) and the stresses of daily life, most of us also need to supplement our diets in some fashion. On a daily basis we are exposed to stress in the form of chemicals, emotions, and infection. Chemical stress may come from polluted air and water, food pesticides, insecticides, heavy metals, and even radioactive wastes. More than ever before, foreign chemicals can be found in our foods and environment. Many of these are commercially synthesized, but quite a few are naturally occurring, as well. In 1989 the Kellogg Report stated that 1,000 newly synthesized compounds are introduced into our environment every year. That's the equivalent of three new chemicals per day. Currently there are approximately 100,000 of these foreign chemicals, or xenobiotics, in the world. They include drugs, pesticides, industrial chemicals, food additives and preservatives, and environmental pollutants. As a result, it's very easy for toxic chemicals to find their way into our bodies via the air we breathe, the foods we eat, and the water we drink. We also ingest these chemicals whenever we use drugs (both medicinal and illicit), alcohol, or tobacco.

Compounding this problem is the fact that the soil in which

our foods are grown is greatly depleted of the trace minerals needed to create and maintain health. Many of our foods are shipped, frozen, stored, and warehoused, reaching us weeks or months after being harvested. Degeneration of their nutrient value occurs at each stop. Cooking methods, such as boiling and frying, also contribute to nutrient loss once the food reaches our kitchens and restaurants. Moreover, the standard American diet has become increasingly devoid of nutrients and overburdened with empty calories and nonfood additives. Therefore, even though the body is marvelously designed to eliminate toxins, in today's environment it needs help in doing so.

Free Radicals and Antioxidants

One of the biggest threats to our health is free radicals, highly toxic molecules that play a causative role in many disease conditions, particularly degenerative disorders such as arthritis, heart disease, cancer, cataracts, macular degeneration, high blood pressure, emphysema, cirrhosis of the liver, ulcers, toxemia during pregnancy, and mental disorders. Free radicals, or oxidants, are very unstable and highly reactive molecules that contain one or more unpaired electrons. They try to capture electrons off other molecules to gain stability, a process known as oxidation. They also increase susceptibility to infection and accelerate the aging process by damaging the cells.

Since free radicals are the primary agents of most cellular damage, minimizing their harmful effects is important. Antioxidants are substances that significantly delay or inhibit oxidation. They neutralize free radicals by supplying electrons. Fortunately, our bodies manufacture antioxidant enzymes within the cells to neutralize and protect against free radicals. Working in tandem with antioxidant nutrients supplied by our diet, such as vitamin A, carotenes, vitamin C, vitamin E, copper, manganese, selenium, and zinc, these enzymes maintain healthy cell function in a variety of ways. As a result, so long as there is an adequate supply of oxygen, water, antioxidant nutrients, and enzymes in the body, cell damage is kept to a minimum. But when our bodies become deficient in any one of these health-enhancing agents, the cells are overrun by free radicals and the antioxidant defenses become unable to maintain their protective shield. This occurs whenever the body's production of antioxidant enzymes and our intake of antioxidant nutrients fall below what is needed to maintain good health. Poor diet, physical and emotional stress, exposure to pollutants, and lack of sleep all contribute to this decline in enzyme production. Escaping such stressors altogether is practically impossible in today's fast-paced world, but help is available in the form of vitamins and other nutritional antioxidant supplements that can offer substantial help in preventing disease, especially arthritis, and maintaining proper immune function.

The following table contains recommended dosages for the most common antioxidant vitamins and minerals, all of which should be part of anyone's daily regimen for creating and maintaining optimal health. Please note that many of general recommendations below are already included in the Arthritis Survival regimen presented on pages 31 to 54. There are a number of multivitamin formulas on the market that contain the ingredients listed below, or you can take them separately. Use the higher dosages whenever you are exposed to higher levels of stress, diminished sleep, increased exposure to pollutants and other sources of toxicity, or when you are not eating as well as you should be. Otherwise take at least the minimum dose every day, preferably with your meals.

RECOMMENDED DAILY NUTRITIONAL SUPPLEMENTS

- **vitamin C (as polyascorbate or Ester-C)**—1,000 to 2,000mg 3 times/day
- **beta-carotene (with mixed carotenoids)**—25,000 IU once or twice a day
- **vitamin E (natural d-alpha mixed tocopherols)**—400 IU once or twice a day
- **B-complex vitamins**—50 to 100mg of each B vitamin per day

- **selenium**—100 to 200mcg per day
- **zinc arginate**—20 to 40mg per day
- **calcium citrate or hydroxyapatite**—1,000mg per day
- **magnesium glycinate or aspartate**—500mg per day
- **chromium polynicotinate (ChromeMate^R)**—200mcg per day
- **manganese**—10 to 15mg per day

In addition to the above, supplementing with *grape-seed extract* (100mg once or twice a day between meals) is also advisable. The antioxidant properties of this supplement has been found to be twenty times greater than vitamin C and fifty times greater than vitamin E.

Daily supplementation of *flaxseed oil, fish oil with EPA/DHA,* and other sources of essential fatty acids are recommended, as well.

Herbal Remedies

Herbs, from which approximately 25 percent of all prescription drugs are derived, have been used for millennia by cultures throughout the world to maintain health and treat and prevent disease. Their proper use is also one of the components of holistic medicine.

While it is not a good idea to employ herbal remedies indiscriminately and without the guidance of a trained practitioner, the following herbs can be safely used by anyone to enhance and maintain health as they generally have a tonic effect and can be taken over a long period of time.

- **Garlic**—A member of the lily family, garlic is a perennial plant cultivated around the world and has been used for thousands of years for its therapeutic properties. Garlic is effective as an antibacterial, antiviral, antifungal, anti-hypertensive, and anti-inflammatory agent; in addition, according to the National Cancer Institute, it shows promise in fighting both stomach and colon cancer. For all of its health-giving properties, however, garlic is also renowned for its distinct odor and the bad breath that it causes. Still, raw garlic, up to a clove a day, is the best way to take it. Otherwise, many brands of processed garlic are now available in pill, capsule, and liquid forms.

- **Cayenne** *(red pepper)*—As a general tonic, cayenne is useful in a variety of ways. It has been shown to increase blood flow and circulation and can help stimulate digestion. According to James Braly, M.D., a specialist in the treatment of food allergies, cayenne can also serve as an anti-inflammatory agent (for used as a topical cream in treating arthritis, see page 55) and can prevent allergic reactions in people with food sensitivities. An excellent way to take cayenne is to use it as a seasoning with your meals. It is also available in capsule form.

- **Ginger**—Ginger has been used medicinally in China and India as far back as the fourth century B.C., primarily to stimulate the gastrointestinal tract and to treat indigestion and flatulence. More recently, ginger has been shown to aid in the treatment of nausea, motion sickness, and coughs and asthma caused by allergy or inflammation. Due to its anti-inflammatory properties, it is also effective in treating arthritis (see page 54). Ginger, along with garlic and onion, has also been found to reduce blood platelet aggregation, indicating that it may be useful in reducing the risk of cardiovascular disease. Ginger can be taken as a tea or in capsule form, and can also be eaten raw and added to meals for flavoring.

- **Echinacea**—Native to the American Midwest, echinacea is a perennial herb renowned for its immune-enhancing properties. In addition to its ability to stimulate the immune system, it is effective as a wound healer, as an antiviral and antibacterial agent, and as an anti-inflammatory. It can be taken alone as a liquid tincture, or in combination with goldenseal, in a dosage of 40 drops taken three times per day. It is also available in capsule form.

According to Steve Morris, N.D., an authority in herbology, echinacea should be regarded as a natural antibiotic. It must be taken regularly in order to have a therapeutic effect, but if taken for periods longer than three weeks, a tolerance to it may occur, thereby negating its effectiveness. Dr. Morris recommends that his patients take the herb daily until their symptoms are completely gone, and then continue for another three to four days to ensure that they do not return. If you choose to use it for longer periods, stop for at least a week following each three-week period of use before resuming again.

- **Ginkgo biloba**—*Ginkgo biloba* is one of the world's oldest living tree species, believed to have survived for 200 million years. In China the ginkgo tree is considered sacred, and in traditional Chinese medicine *Ginkgo biloba* is commonly prescribed for respiratory ailments and to maintain and improve brain function. *Ginkgo* has been shown to increase circulation to the brain and is therefore helpful with dementia, Alzheimer's disease, memory loss, concentration problems, vertigo, tinnitus, and dizziness. It can also be used in cases of peripheral vascular disease, such as Raynaud's syndrome, intermittent claudication (severe pain in the calf muscle brought about by walking), numbness, and tingling. Studies have also reported *ginkgo*'s usefulness in improving cases of head injury, macular degeneration, asthma, and impotence. The usual daily dose is 120 milligrams.

Food Allergy

Food allergy ranks as one of the most common conditions in the United States. Compounding this problem is the fact that millions of Americans are unaware that they are having negative reactions to the foods they eat. Ironically, the foods to which we react are the foods we crave the most. The foods that most commonly cause allergy are cow's milk and all dairy products, wheat and other grains, chocolate, corn, sugar, soy, yeast (both brewer's and baker's), oranges, tomatoes, bell peppers, white potatoes, eggs, fish, shellfish, cocoa, onions, nuts, garlic, peanuts, black pepper, red meat, coffee, black tea, and beer, wine, and champagne. Aspirin and artificial food colorings can also cause allergic reactions. But as holistic physicians know, any substance can cause an unsuspected allergic reaction, even water.

Doris Rapp, M.D., past president of the American Academy of Environmental Medicine and author of *Allergies and Your Family,* recommends the following method for detecting food allergies. Take your pulse in the morning, on an empty stomach. Count your heartbeat for a full minute. Then eat the food you wish to test. Wait fifteen to thirty minutes, then retake your pulse. If your heart rate has increased by fifteen to twenty beats per minute, chances are that you are sensitive to the food you ate. You may also want to consider food allergy testing as previously mentioned through Great Smokies Laboratory (see Resource Guide).

The symptoms of food allergy are many and usually occur within four days after eating the food in question, further contributing to the fact that food allergies are often overlooked as an underlying cause of poor health. *In the case of joint effects, the symptoms can take seven to twelve days to appear.* Nearly every organ system of the body can be the target of food reactions, including the brain (foggy-headedness), heart (rhythm distrubances), lungs (asthma), gastrointestinal tract (ulcers, colitis), veins (phlebitis), bladder (frequency, urgency, enuresis), and joints (arthritis). If you suspect you suffer from food allergies, consult a holistic physician or practitioner of environmental medicine, who offers a more comprehensive perspective on allergies and food sensitivities than more conventional allergy specialists do. To find such a physician in your area, contact The American Academy of Environmental Medicine at (316) 684-5500.

Exercise and Physical Activity

No discussion of physical health would be complete without including the subject of exercise and physical activity. Regular exercise can contribute more to optimal health than any other health practice, with the possible exception of diet. Yet, in spite of exercise's many proven benefits, we are becoming an increasingly sedentary nation. This is especially true of our children, who are becoming fatter (25 percent are overweight), weaker, and slower than ever before.

Numerous studies show that sedentary people, on average, don't live as long or enjoy as good health as those who get regular aerobic exercise in the form of brisk walking, running, swimming, cycling, rebounding (jumping on a mini-trampoline), or similar workouts. In fact, some researchers now believe that lack of exercise may be a more significant risk factor for decreased life expectancy than the *combined* risks of cigarette smoking, high cholesterol, being overweight, and high blood pressure. Simply put, *being unfit means being unhealthy.*

The benefits of regular exercise and physical activity include dissipation of tension; decreased "fight or flight" response, depression, anxiety, smoking, drug use, and incidence of heart disease and cancer; increased self-esteem, a more positive attitude, and greater joy, spontaneity, mental acuity, mental function, aerobic capacity, and enhanced energy; increased muscular strength and flexibility; and improved quality of sleep. Regular exercise also results in increased lean/fat ratio and increased longevity (people who are least fit have a mortality rate 3.5 times as great as those who are most fit).

Some of the more pronounced benefits of regular exercise occur with older women. A seven-year study conducted by the University of Minnesota School of Public Health tracked the physical activity levels of over 40,000 women, all of whom were postmenopausal and ranged in age from 55 to 69. The results showed that women who exercised at least four times a week at high intensity had up to a 30-percent lowered risk of early death as compared to women in the same age group who were sedentary. But even infrequent (once a week) exercisers among participants in the study experienced reduced mortality rates.

In selecting an exercise program, choose a blend of activities that will increase *aerobic capacity, strength, and flexibility* and refer to the exercise recommendations on page 58. You'll want to choose an exercise program that is easy on your joints. A regimen focused solely on strength conditioning, such as weight lifting, while providing strength, does little to increase aerobic capacity and can even diminish flexibility. Adding a stretching routine and an aerobic workout on alternate days will provide a much more effective exercise practice.

Breathing

We can live for weeks without food and days without water, but if we stop breathing for more than two or three minutes, we die. Breathing is the single most important physical function we perform; yet, almost all of us breathe inefficiently. For the most part, we aren't even conscious of our breath, and spend hour after hour breathing shallowly into the chest, depriving ourselves of the tremendous energy and revitalizing power that proper breathing can provide.

The primary purpose of breathing is to deliver oxygen to every cell in every tissue and organ in the body while removing carbon dioxide. Oxygen's primary role in the body is to produce the energy required for every basic bodily function via its interaction with adenosine triphosphate (ATP). Since the cellular content of ATP is responsible for the body's total energy levels and its ability to perform all of its functions, adequate oxygen levels are essential for our overall health. When our oxygen intake is reduced, ATP is diminished as well.

A variety of environmental factors can also contribute to oxygen deficiency, including high carbon monoxide and smoke pollution, smog, and high altitude. (Oxygen content decreases by over 3 percent every thousand feet above sea level.) The primary cause of chronic reduced oxygen levels in the body, however, is due to shallow and inefficient breathing patterns. Typically, most of us habitually breathe in through the chest, failing to breathe deeply and fully. This unconscious and inefficient method of breathing significantly reduces our oxygen supply. By simply learning how to improve the way you breathe, you can considerably improve your health and ensure that your cells remain in an oxygen-rich state.

Practice abdominal breathing. Breathing through the abdomen instead of through the chest is a simple yet powerful way to improve energy and flow of oxygen, enhance digestion, relieve stomach pain and flatulence, and diminish stress. Since most of us rarely breathe through our bellies, learning to do so at first may seem odd. Yet, abdominal breathing is easy to do. Just direct your breath in and out through your belly. If you do so correctly, your chest will not move. You can easily check this by placing one hand on your belly and the other on your chest. As you breathe, the lower hand should move, while the hand on your chest should remain motionless.

Don't get discouraged if you are unable to accomplish this on your first try. Make it a practice to spend a few minutes each day breathing abdominally (working up to twenty to thirty minutes a day is recommended), along with regular brief sessions whenever you notice yourself feeling tense or irritable. Abdominal breathing can also be performed in conjunction with meditation (see page 170).

Do your best to breathe clean, moist, negative-ion, and oxygen-rich air, both at home and at work. Refer to the environmental health section at the end of this chapter.

Aerobic Exercise

The word *aerobic* means "with oxygen." Aerobic exercise refers to prolonged exercise that requires extra oxygen to supply energy to the muscles. In general, aerobic activities cause moderate shortness of breath, perspiring, and doubling of the resting pulse rate. A few words of conversation should be possible at the height of activity; otherwise the workout may in fact be too strenuous.

Aerobic exercise is determined by maintaining your *target heart rate,* which produces greater benefits to the cardiovascular system and provides more oxygen to the body than any other form of exercise. To determine what your target heart rate should be, use the following formula: 220 minus your age, multiplied by 60 to 85 percent. Keep in mind that 60 percent is considered low intensity or *mild* aerobic exercise, with 70 percent being *moderate,* and 85 percent being high intensity or *strenuous.* For example, a 40-year-old's target heart rate is between 108 and 153 beats per minute. To accurately determine your pulse, use your index and middle finger to feel the pulse on the thumb side of your wrist or at your neck, just below the jaw. Using a watch with a secondhand, count the number of beats in 60 seconds (or 15 seconds and multiply by 4), which will give you your heart rate in beats per minute.

When you have attained your target heart rate (after about five to ten minutes of exercising), try to maintain it for at least twenty minutes. It is also beneficial to cool down by working out at a slower heart rate and with less intensity for an additional five to ten minutes before you end your session.

The most convenient forms of aerobic exercise involving the least amount of wear and tear on the body are brisk walking, hiking, swimming, rebounding, and cycling. Cross-country skiing, if convenient, can also provide a very good aerobic workout. These are all good choices while healing arthritic joints. Jogging can also be effective, but due to the rising number of patients with running-related complaints, it is recommended that you stretch thoroughly before and after each run, use good running shoes and orthotics (if indicated), and supplement your diet with vitamin C and calcium to strengthen your bones, cartilage, muscles, and tendons. If your arthritis is in your knees, hips, or spine, I recommend that you avoid jogging. Treadmills, rowing machines, stair climbers, and cross-country ski machines also offer an opportunity for excellent indoor aerobics, as do low-impact aerobics classes. Racquetball, handball, badminton, singles tennis, and basketball provide good aerobic workouts as well. But these are also high-impact activities that someone who is healing an arthritic knee or hip should participate in very cautiously at first.

The keys to a successful aerobic routine are consistency and comfort. Aerobic conditioning does not have to entail a great deal of time, nor does it have to be painful. Find an activity that you can enjoy without any joint pain, and keep it fun. Remember, too, that low to moderate aerobic exercise for forty-five minutes is just as beneficial as high-intensity exercise for twenty minutes. Exercise outdoors whenever possible, as long as it is convenient and safe to do so, as the combination of fresh air and sunshine provides greater health benefits than does indoor exercise.

Caution: *Do not begin any aerobic activity in the heat of an emotional crisis, especially intense anger.* Wait at least 15 to 20 minutes to avoid the risk of heart attack or arrhythmias that can be triggered under such circumstances. In addition, make sure your aerobic exercise precedes meals by at least half an hour, or follows them by at least two and a half hours, in order to avoid indigestion.

Strength Conditioning

Building and maintaining muscle strength is another essential component to your overall exercise program. Strength conditioning falls under three categories: *(1) strengthening without aids,* which includes calisthenics such as sit-ups, push-ups, jumping jacks, and swimming; *(2) strengthening with aids,* which includes chin-ups, dips, weight lifting, and training on weight machines; and *(3) strengthening with aerobics,* which involves various forms of interval training that can be done in association with running, bicycling, jumping rope, circuit training with weight machines, and working out on a heavy bag. The goal of interval training is to work intensively, reaching your maximum heart level for a short interval; then lower the level of activity to recover. Repeating this process while maintaining your heart rate in its target zone reduces recovery time, strengthens various muscle groups, and conditions the cardiovascular system.

Weight training is perhaps the most popular form of strength conditioning exercise. To design a weight program to meet your specific needs, consult with a personal trainer, who will most likely advise you to work out two or three times a week. It isn't necessary to lift a lot of weight to build and tone muscle. If muscle tone and definition is your goal, best results will be achieved using less weight and more repetitions. To build mass, increase the amount of weight you use and do fewer repetitions. Remember to breathe out as you exert effort, and for free-weight exercises it is advisable to work with a spotter. Also wear a weight belt to help keep your spine properly aligned.

Increasing Flexibility

The final component of a good exercise program addresses flexibility. This includes stretching exercises, yoga, tai chi, and the Feldenkrais Method. Exercise that promotes flexibility also significantly contributes to strength and function by allowing the body's muscle groups to perform at maximum efficiency. It also enhances blood flow, which in turn helps to maintain healthy joints. Lack of flexibility can restrict blood flow, severely inhibit physical performance, increase the potential for injury, and compromise posture. Muscles exist in a state of static tension wherein contrasting sets of muscles exert similar force to create a state of balance. When muscles become weak or inflexible, this balance is disrupted, resulting in reduced function or postural misalignment. Additional benefits of muscle flexibility include enhanced suppleness of connective tissue (fascia, tendons, and ligaments) and greater body awareness.

Stretching exercises. Some form of stretching is recommended before and after both aerobic and strengthening workouts. Before you begin stretching, do five minutes of movement to warm up your muscles and body core. This will enhance your circulation and make stretching easier. Never stretch to the point of pain. Ideally, you should feel a tension in the affected muscle or muscle group that you are working. As you do, breathe into the stretch to elongate and relax the muscle group as you hold the posture for twenty to thirty seconds. Repeat each stretch at least twice. You should notice that your range increases on the second and third repetition. A few minutes of daily stretching will noticeably improve your well-being over time. Both yoga and tai chi are excellent forms of exercise for helping to heal arthritic joints. The Feldenkrais Method is described on page 74.

Yoga. Yoga is a Sanskrit word meaning "to yoke" and refers to a balanced practice of physical exercise, breathing, and meditation to unify body, mind, and spirit, making yoga one of the most effective and ancient forms of holistic self-care. The benefits of this five-thousand-year-old system of mind/body training to improve flexibility, strength, and concentration are well documented. There are a number of yogic systems, with *hatha yoga* being most well known in the West. Hatha yoga postures, or *asanas,* affect specific muscle groups and organs to impart physical strength and flexibility as well as emotional and mental peace of mind.

There are a variety of hatha yoga forms available. Initially it is a good idea to receive instruction for at least a few months, due to the subtleties involved in yoga practice that are not apparent without firsthand experience under the guidance of a qualified yoga instructor.

Tai chi chuan. Sometimes referred to as "meditation in motion," tai chi, like yoga, is thousands of years old and involves slow motion movements integrated with focused breathing and visualization. Practiced daily by tens of millions of people in the People's Republic of China, the goal of tai chi is to move *qi* ("chee") or "vital life-force energy" along the various meridians, or energetic pathways, of the body's various organ systems. According to traditional Chinese medicine, when the flow of *qi* is balanced and unobstructed, both blood and lymph flow are enhanced and the body's neurological impulses function at optimal capacity. The result is greater vitality, resistance to disease, stimulation of the "relaxation response," increased oxygenation of the blood, deeper sleep, and increased body/mind awareness. Although not as well known as yoga in this country, tai chi is rapidly gaining in popularity and tai chi instructors can be found in most metropolitan areas. After being taught the basic movements of tai chi, you can practice them almost anywhere to instill a centeredness and sense of calm that is a proven method of alleviating stress.

Sleep and Relaxation

While diet, the use of supplements, and exercise can all benefit physical health and improve immune function, perhaps the most powerful and often overlooked key to overall well-being is sleep. The average person requires between eight and nine hours of uninterrupted sleep; yet, in the U.S. we average between six and eight hours, with an estimated 50 million Americans suffering from insomnia.

Lack of sleep and its resulting depression of the immune system can be a factor in many chronic health conditions including arthritis, and is a common cause of colds. Additional sleep is therefore an essential component in the holistic treatment of any such conditions. Besides lowered immune function, sleep deprivation can also cause a decrease in productivity, creativity, and job performance, and can affect mood and mental alertness. In cases of insomnia, most incidents of sleep deprivation are due to a specific stress-producing event. While stress-induced insomnia is usually temporary, it may persist well beyond the precipitating event to become a chronic problem. Overstimulation of the nervous system (especially due to caffeine, salt, or sugar), or simply the fear that you can't fall asleep, are other common causes.

Researchers have identified two types of sleep: *heavy* and *light*. During heavier, or nonrapid-eye-movement (NREM) sleep, your body's self-healing mechanisms are revitalized, enabling your body to repair itself. During lighter, rapid-eye-movement (REM) sleep, you dream more, releasing stress and tension. (For more on dreams, see Chapter 5.)

Conventional medicine commonly prescribes sleeping pills for insomnia and other sleep disorders, but as with almost all medications, there are unpleasant side effects to contend with, as well as the risk of developing dependency. A more holistic approach to ensuring adequate sleep begins with establishing a regular bedtime every night so that you can begin to re-attune yourself to nature's rhythms. According to Ayurvedic medicine (see page 70), the circadian rhythm, caused by the earth rotating on its axis every twenty-four hours, has a counterpart in the human body. Modern science has confirmed that many neurological and endocrine functions follow this circadian rhythm, including the sleep-wakefulness cycle. Ayurveda teaches that the ideal bedtime for the deepest sleep and for being in sync with this natural rhythm is 10 P.M. Unfortunately, most people with insomnia dread bedtime and go to bed later, when sleep tends to be somewhat lighter and more active. Ayurveda also states that eight hours of sleep beginning at 9:30 P.M. is twice as restful as eight hours beginning at 2 A.M. It is also important in resetting your biological clock to get up early and at the same time every day, regardless of when you go to bed. Establishing an early wake-up time (6 or 7 A.M.) is essential for overcoming insomina. You'll eventually begin to feel sleepier earlier in the evening, and even if you aren't actually sleeping by 10 P.M., you'll bene-fit just by resting in bed at that hour.

Most importantly, don't worry about lost sleep, since in most cases anxiety is what caused the problem in the first place. If you can learn to relax without drugs, you will have cured your sleep-ing problems while giving your immune system a powerful boost.

Relaxation is another essential ability that promotes physical health. Derived from the Latin *relaxare,* meaning "to loosen," re-laxation is a way to allow the mind to return to a natural state of equilibrium, creating a state of balance between the right and left brain. It is also a highly effective means of stress reduction.

Relaxation is a skill that can be improved upon with practice; therefore it is recommended that you take time each day to relax. This can be achieved as easily as taking a few deep breaths or simply shifting your focus away from your problems and con-cerns, or through any activity that engages your creative and physical faculties. Such activities include reading and writing, gardening, taking a walk, painting, singing, playing music, mak-ing crafts, or doing any other hobby that you enjoy for its own sake, without the need to be concerned about your perfor-mance. Committing two to three evening hours a week to the hobby or activity of your choice will help make relaxation a natural and regular part of your daily experience. The ability to relax and shift gears away from the competitive drive that compels most of us in our society holds the key to greater health.

Environmental Medicine

COMPONENTS OF OPTIMAL ENVIRONMENTAL HEALTH

Harmony with your environment (neither harming nor being harmed)
- awareness of your connectedness with nature
- feeling grounded—comfort and securtiy within your surroundings
- respect and appreciation for your home, the Earth, and all of her inhabitants;
- contact with the earth; breathing healthy air; drinking pure water; eating uncontaminated food; exposure to the sun, fire, or candlelight; immersion in warm water (all on a daily basis).

As discussed above, our environment is increasingly becoming burdened with a proliferation of toxic chemicals and pollutants. Environmental medicine deals with these environmental hazards as well as communicable diseases and the potential health risks that are becoming increasingly common in work and social settings. The modern-day roots of environmental medicine go back to the late 1940's and the work of Theron G. Randolph, M.D., one of the first physicians to notice the negative impact that chemicals in the environment could have on the body. Today, Dr. Randolph's work is primarily carried on by the American Academy of Environmental Medicine (AAEM) (see Resource Guide). This organization trains physicians in treating illnesses caused by environmental factors.

The range of diseases that have been linked to the environment is both extensive and growing. The body systems affected include the immune, cardiovascular, respiratory, endocrine, gastrointestinal, nervous, genitourinary, and musculoskeletal. Environmental factors also play a role in many pediatric diseases; eyes, nose, ear, and throat conditions; skin conditions; and mental illness, and have also been linked to certain forms of cancer. Among the elements that can contribute to environmentally caused illness are poor nutrition and diet, stress, air- and water-borne chemical exposure, infection, heredity and genetic predisposition, dental mercury amalgam fillings, the overuse of antibiotics and other medications, glandular and hormonal imbalances, and electromagnetic radiation.

Like food allergies, environmental illness is often undiagnosed. If you suspect that environmental factors may be impacting your health, contact the AAEM for a referral to a physician in your area. Overall, professional guidance is usually required to deal with serious cases of environmental illness, but there are also a variety of self-care measures that you can use preventively and therapeutically. Hal Huggins, D.D.S., a leader in the field of biological dentistry, has found that symptoms of arthritis are often associated with dental mercury amalgam fillings. He notes that once the amalgams are removed, the symptoms usually disappear.

Nothing is more important to our health than the air we breathe. The healthiest air is clean, moist, warm, and high in both oxygen and negative ion content. According to the Environmental Protection Agency (EPA), however, 60 percent of all Americans live in areas where poor air quality is a health risk. An additional detriment lies in the adverse effects that many newer, air-conditioned buildings and office spaces can have in the form of "sick-building syndrome." Researchers in France, for instance, have found that workers in such indoor environments are twice as likely to suffer from respiratory problems as people who work outdoors or in buildings without air-conditioning. Moreover, the researchers' findings indicate that such buildings are breeding grounds for airborne bacteria and fungi and contribute to a greater incidence of asthma, colds, sinus infections, runny noses, and sore throats. Compounding this problem is the fact that the majority of Americans spend 90 percent of their time inside, where, according to the EPA, the air can be as much as one hundred times more polluted than outdoor air.

To safeguard against the harmful effects of bad air and other environmental factors, supplement your diet with antioxidants, especially if you live in a city. Proper diet and good drinking water are also essential. Creating a setting of indoor plants where you work and at home can also be helpful. Not only do plants oxygenate the air and create more moisture, they also filter out carbon monoxide and organic chemicals, add beauty to the environment, and can enhance feelings of well-being. Also consider the use of a negative-ion generator and humidifier.

Negative ions, which are air molecules containing an excess of electrons, can substantially vitalize the air we breathe. Studies have shown that negative ions increase the sweeping motion of the cilia on the respiratory mucosa, thereby enhancing the movement of mucus and the expulsion and filtration of inhaled pollutants. They also help reduce pain, heal burns, suppress mold and bacteria, and stimulate plant growth. Positive ions, by contrast, have an opposite effect and are largely the by-product of man-made pollutants, such as auto and truck exhaust, smokestacks, and cigarette smoke. Heating and filtration systems also tend to produce air high in positive-ion content, as do window air conditioners, air cleaners (including HEPA filters), television sets, and computer monitors. Airplane cabins contain an inordinate amount of positive ions, as well. The use of a negative ion generator can significantly increase negative ion content in an indoor environment, minimizing positive ion effects.

Dry air, especially if it is cold, is also harmful to health and is quite common in many modern buildings. Dry air is a major contributor to sinusitis and chronic bronchitis and is also a factor in allergies. Optimum indoor air quality contains 35 to 55 percent relative humidity, which can easily be achieved by using a room humidifier. Humidifiers are particularly useful in the winter months, because most heating systems dry the indoor air considerably. Of the variety of room humidifiers available, warm-mist units are most effective. These produce a mist just slightly warmer than room air, use tap water, require no filter, and are able to kill bacteria. Be sure to clean them at least weekly with vinegar. Their only limitation is that they also tend to require more electricity than other models.

Another important strategy for minimizing indoor environmental pollution is the use of materials that emit no pollutants. Natural products such as wood, cotton, and metals are preferable to synthetic materials such as particleboard, fiberboard, polyester, and plastics. Synthetic carpets are also high in potentially toxic ingredients. Beware of formaldehyde from insulation materials, unpainted particleboard, and plywood as well. Substitutes of cellulose and white fiberglass insulation are recommended. Cleaning substances can also be a source of indoor pollution, due to their chemical content. In their place, use nontoxic substances, including ordinary soap, vinegar, and zephiran.

Other self-care steps you can take to protect yourself from environmental pollution include:

* avoiding secondhand tobacco smoke
* using highly efficient furnace filters in your home
* reducing usage of coal- or wood-burning fireplaces and stoves
* sleeping with your bedroom window open to ensure a stream of fresh air
* taking frequent breaks away from your computer
* making a habit of spending regular periods of time outdoors in an unpolluted, natural setting
* moving to a healthier neighborhood or city
* cleaning carpets and rugs regularly with nontoxic cleaners to prevent buildup of mold and bacteria
* ensuring that both your home and workplace benefit from good ventilation.

Becoming environmentally healthy requires conscious attention and effort. Remember, environmental health is a condition of respect and appreciation for your home, community, nature, and the Earth. It is a relationship of harmony with your environment so that you are enhanced and enlivened by your surroundings instead of harming or being harmed by them. The more that you become involved in improving the conditions of your environment, the healthier you will be.

Summary

Committing yourself to a consistent program of eating well, taking the proper supplements, becoming more physically fit,

and creating a healthy environment based on the recommendations in this chapter will enable you to achieve improvements in
your physical well-being in as little as a few weeks. You may also
notice significant improvement in the condition of your joints,
but be aware that with arthritis you'll need to progress more
gradually. Before long, you will find that your reserves of energy
are greater and that you are physically stronger, more powerful,
and more flexible. You will also develop a more positive self-
image and feel better about how your body looks and performs
in every realm of activity. And if you have been spending more
time outdoors, you will feel more connected to and empowered
by nature.

Optimal physical health is a feeling of *harmony* within your
body. It will be experienced as an *effortless flowing of all bodily
functions and fluids.* Your breathing will become more abdominal
and less restricted, providing a greater supply of oxygen to every
cell as it flows through less constricted arteries. Enhanced by an
increased intake of water, your circulation will in turn allow
your kidneys and bowels more complete elimination of toxins
and waste. Your more nutritious diet will provide better nourishment and more energy to your cells. And your more regular
and effortless bowel movements will be more conducive to
maximum absorption of nutrients. Your body movement and
exercise programs will even further facilitate the nourishment of
all cells, tissues, and organs.

As you begin to thrive, you will be sleeping more deeply and
making time for relaxation. You will enjoy greater sexual energy
and often greater endurance and pleasure. You will become
more aware and appreciative of the miracle of your own body,
and the intelligence and efficiency with which it regulates and
heals itself. You will also have a better understanding of how
your body relates to and is impacted by the environment surrounding it. You may even develop a sense of how the improved
harmony with your environment may enhance your longevity.

Your body is simply working better. As a result, it can provide
you with some of life's simplest but greatest pleasures: deep
sleep, uncongested breathing, graceful movement, unrestricted

urination, easy bowel movements, fulfilling sexual intercourse, and an awareness of the unimpeded flow of life energy that connects us to one another and to our environment. Such benefits are just the beginning of your journey to optimal well-being. They will continue to become more noticeable as you take more responsibility for your health and follow this chapter's guidelines in the months and years ahead. In the process, you will be creating the foundation necessary for healing the other aspects of holistic medicine's triumvirate—*mind and spirit*—while you are healing your degenerative joint dis-ease.

Chapter 5

HEALING YOUR MIND

"The greatest discovery of any generation is that human beings can alter their lives by altering the attitudes of their minds."

ALBERT SCHWEITZER

COMPONENTS OF OPTIMAL MENTAL HEALTH

Peace of mind and contentment

- A job that you love doing
- Optimism
- A sense of humor
- Financial well-being
- Living your life vision.
- The ability to express your creativity and talents
- The capacity to make healthy decisions

COMPONENTS OF OPTIMAL EMOTIONAL HEALTH

Self-acceptance and high self-esteem

- The capacity to identify, express, experience, and accept all of your feelings, both painful and joyful
- Awareness of the intimate connection between your physical and emotional bodies
- The ability to confront your greatest fears
- The fulfillment of your capacity to play
- Peak experiences on a regular basis.

One of the most exciting developments in the field of medicine in recent decades has been the scientific verification that our physical health is directly influenced by our thoughts and emotions. The reverse is also true: Overwhelming evidence now exists showing that our physiology has a direct correlation to the ways we habitually think and feel. While eastern systems of medicine, such as traditional Chinese medicine and Ayurveda, have for centuries recognized these facts and stressed the importance of a harmonious connection between body and mind, in the West this mind-body connection did not begin to be acknowledged until research conducted in the 1970s and '80s conclusively revealed the ability of thoughts, emotions, and attitudes to influence our bodies' immune functions. In fact, many of the scientists exploring this relatively new field have concluded that **there is no separation between mind and body.**

In order to heal our minds and emotions, it helps to know what we mean by the term *mental health.* From the perspective of holistic medicine, the essence of mental health is peace of mind and feelings of contentment. Being mentally healthy means that you recognize the ways in which your thoughts, beliefs, mental imagery, and attitudes affect your well-being and limit or expand your ability to enjoy your life. It also means knowing that you always have choices about what you think and believe, and are aware of your gifts, are practicing your special talents, working at a job that you enjoy, and being clear about your priorities, values, and goals. People who have made a commitment to their mental health live their lives with rich reserves of humor and optimism. They have chosen a nurturing set of beliefs and attitudes that fills them with peace and hope. Most people who buy this book do so with the belief, however minimal, that they do not have to suffer with arthritis for the rest of their lives. Since you have read to this point and begun practicing the physical components of the Arthritis Survival Program, your belief has probably been strengthened considerably. You can determine your own state of mental health by referring to the appropriate section of the Wellness Self-Test at the end of Chapter 3, and then use the information in this chapter to improve the areas you may need to work on.

The term *mental health* can be interpreted to include not only our thoughts and beliefs but also our feelings. However, when your focus is specifically on "feelings," this is the realm of *emotional health*. These aspects of ourselves—**mental** and **emotional**—are for the most part inextricably related and together form the "**mind**" aspect of holistic health. As your healing journey progresses, you will increasingly come to recognize how your own distorted or illogical thoughts are the underlying cause of feelings such as anger, depression, anxiety, fear, and unfounded guilt. Learning how to free yourself from such distorted thinking patterns is the goal of this chapter, and of behavioral medicine, the aspect of holistic medicine that deals with this interconnectedness between physical, mental, and emotional health. Behavioral medicine includes professional treatment approaches such as *psychotherapy, mind/body medicine, guided imagery and visualization, biofeedback therapy, hypnotherapy, neurolinguistic programming (NLP), orthomolecular medicine* (the use of nutritional supplements to treat chronic mental disease), *flower essences,* and *body-centered therapies like Rolfing and Hellerwork* (these two therapies which can also be quite helpful in treating arthritis are described in Chapter 4).

However, with the exception of psychotherapy, the focus in this chapter is on proven self-care approaches that you can begin using immediately to heal the mind along with your painful joints. They include *creating new beliefs and establishing clear goals, affirmations, breathwork, guided imagery, visualization, meditation, dreamwork, journaling,* and *your approaches to both work and play*. Each of these methods can help you become more aware of your habitual thoughts, attitudes, and emotions—both pleasurable and painful—in order to create a mind-set conducive to experiencing optimal health and more effectively meeting your professional goals and personal desires, including freeing yourself from the pain of arthritis.

THE BODY–MIND CONNECTION

Growing numbers of western scientists and physicians now recognize that *body* and *mind* are not separate aspects of our being but interrelated expressions of the same experience. Their view is based on the findings of researchers working in the field of *psychoneuroimmunology (PNI)*, also referred to as *neuroscience,* which for the past three decades has shown us that our thoughts, emotions, and attitudes can directly influence immune and hormone function. In light of such research, scientists now commonly speak of the mind's ability to control the body. In large part, this perspective is due to the scientific discovery of "messenger" molecules known as *neuropeptides,* chemicals that communicate our thoughts, emotions, attitudes, and beliefs to every cell in our body. In practical terms, this means that all of us are capable of both weakening or strengthening our immune systems according to how we think and feel. Moreover, scientists have also proven that these messages can originate not only in the brain but from every cell in our body. As a result of such studies, scientists now conclude that the immune system actually functions as a "circulating nervous system" that is actively and acutely attuned to our every thought and emotion.

Among the discoveries which have occurred in the field of PNI are the following:

- Feelings of loss and self-rejection can diminish immune function and contribute to a number of chronic disease conditions, including heart attack.
- Feelings of exhilaration and joy produce measurable levels of a neuropeptide identical to interleukin-2, a powerful anti-cancer drug that costs many thousands of dollars per injection.
- Feelings of peace and calm produce a chemical very similar to Valium, a popular tranquillizer.
- Depressive states negatively impact the immune system and increase the likelihood of illness.
- Chronic grief or a sense of loss can increase the likelihood of cancer.

- Anxiety and fear can trigger high blood pressure.
- Feelings of hostility, grief, depression, hopelessness, and isolation greatly increase the risk of heart attack.
- Repressed anger is a factor in causing many chronic ailments, including sinusitis, bronchitis, headaches, and candidiasis.
- Acknowledgment and expression of feelings strengthens immune responses.
- Anger decreases immunoglobulin A (a protective antibody) in saliva, while caring, compassion, humor, and laughter increase it.
- Chronic stress has a broad suppressive effect on immunity, including the depression of natural killer cells, which attack cancer cells.

As exciting as these discoveries are, the studies that had the greatest impact on me were performed on multiple-personality patients at the National Institutes of Health (NIH). Scientists found that in one personality an individual could have the strongest possible skin reaction to an allergen or be severely nearsighted, but after shifting to another personality (an unconscious process in the *same* body) there was *no skin reaction* to the same allergen and perfectly normal *20/20 vision!* Science is just beginning to understand the depth and power of the connection between mind and body.

The implications of these discoveries are enormous and are producing a paradigmatic shift in physicians' approaches to treating chronic disease. They play an essential role in the Arthritis Survival Program: If emotions and attitudes can contribute to causing heart disease and cancer, it isn't too difficult to appreciate how they can also play a role in arthritis. They are also tremendously empowering for anyone committed to holistic health. Once you accept the fact that there is an ongoing, instant, and intimate communication occurring between your mind and your body via the mechanisms of neuropeptides, you can also see that the person best qualified to direct that communication in your own life is you. Learning how to do so effectively can enable you to become your own 24-hours-a-day healer by becoming more conscious of your thoughts and emotions and managing them better to improve all areas of your health. The first step in this process is acknowledging that you can no longer afford to continue feeding yourself the same limiting messages you most likely have been conditioned to accept since early childhood. Scientists now estimate that the average person has approximately fifty-thousand thoughts each day; yet, 95 percent of them are the same as the ones he or she had the day before. Typically such thoughts are not only unconscious but often critical and limiting. For example, "I'll never be able to overcome this arthritis [or any chronic illness]." "I may not be capable of caring for myself, and I'll become a burden on my family." "I'm going to have to live with this pain and suffering for the rest of my life." When you're hearing messages like these repeated many times during the course of a typical day, it's easy to understand why for most people with a chronic condition like arthritis, *fear, anger, hopelessness, sadness,* and *depression* may become their predominant feelings. You've just read that these painful emotions can be associated with weakening the immune system while also contributing to a myriad of physical problems. Degenerative joint disease is no exception. However, *by consciously taking control of your thoughts and recognizing how they govern your behavior, you can dramatically change your life and heal your dis-ease.* You will gain the freedom to think, feel, and believe as you choose, thereby flooding your body's cells with positive, life-affirming messages capable of producing optimal health. I've described this condition as the unlimited and unimpeded free flow of life force energy through your body, mind, and spirit. The remainder of this chapter provides a variety of approaches to enhance this flow of life energy through your mind.

PSYCHOTHERAPY

The field of psychotherapy, an outgrowth of the theories and discoveries of Sigmund Freud, continues to evolve more than a hundred years since its inception. In addition to the mental and emotional benefits commonly attributed to psychotherapy, a growing body of research has documented that physical benefits can also occur. For example, in a study conducted at the UCLA School of Medicine by the late Norman Cousins, a group of cancer patients receiving psychotherapy for ninety minutes a week showed dramatic improvement in their immune systems after only six weeks. During that same period the control group of other cancer patients who received no counseling showed no change in immune function whatsoever.

Psychotherapy, by its very nature, is not a self-care protocol but can be extremely valuable for individuals struggling with deep-rooted mental and emotional problems. *The most popular forms of psychotherapy are classical or Freudian psychoanalysis, Jungian psychoanalysis, family therapy, cognitive/behavioral therapy, brief/ solution-focused therapy, and humanistic/existential therapy. Though they all share the same goal of helping patients achieve mental health, their approaches can vary widely.*

If you feel that psychotherapy may help you, you will gain the most benefit by choosing the approach best suited to your specific needs and objectives. In addition, be aware that the work of psychotherapy is increasingly being conducted by non-psychiatrists, including psychologists, social workers, and pastoral counselors. One of the reasons for this, perhaps, lies in the fact that many of today's patients seeing psychiatrists are given a psychiatric diagnosis (depression, manic-depressive, obsessive-compulsive, etc.) and then treated with drugs, such as the anti-depressant Prozac. This trend within psychiatry, a departure away from counseling toward greater drug therapy, makes it a less desirable choice for someone interested in a holistic and self-care approach. While psychotherapeutic drugs can be effective at times, especially over the short term, each of the drugs commonly prescribed by psychiatrists has the potential to cause unpleasant side effects. Equally important, by focusing on treating psychological symptoms with drugs, many psychiatrists are depriving their patients of the opportunity to change their attitudes and behavior and to learn how to understand and grow from their emotional pain. Finally, whichever type of psychotherapist you choose, make sure that he or she is someone with whom you are comfortable. Psychotherapy can only be effective in a situation of trust, so you may wish to interview a number of therapists before making your choice.

BELIEFS, ATTITUDES, GOALS, AND AFFIRMATIONS

In his classic treatise *The Science of Mind,* noted spiritual teacher Ernest Holmes wrote: "Health and sickness are largely externalizations of our dominant mental and spiritual states. A normal healthy mind reflects itself in a healthy body, and conversely, an abnormal mental state expresses its corresponding condition in some physical condition." At the time Holmes wrote those words, in the mid-1920's, modern science was far behind him in understanding how *our thoughts directly influence our physical health.* But today a growing body of evidence not only verifies this fact but also indicates that it is our predominant, habitual beliefs that determine the thoughts we primarily think. Socrates stated that the unexamined life was not worth living. Based on today's research in the field of behavioral medicine, we may paraphrase his statement to say, *"The unexamined belief is not worth believing in."* Yet, most of us have never taken the time to actually examine the beliefs we hold, and therefore remain unaware of how they may be influencing our well-being.

The importance of beliefs in the overall scheme of human functioning is confirmed by placebo studies. A placebo is a dummy medication or procedure possessing no therapeutic properties that works only because of our belief in it. Detailed analysis of thirteen placebo studies from 1940 to 1979, including 1,200 patients, found an 82 percent improvement resulting from the use of medications or procedures that subsequently proved to be placebos.

Changing your beliefs is essential to your success with the Arthritis Survival Program. Many people suffering with arthritis have been told by their physicians: "You're going to have to live with this problem"; "The only thing that can be done is to take anti-inflammatory medication to relieve the pain"; "Eventually you'll need to have a knee or hip replacement"; or "There's nothing more that can be done for your arthritis [or the majority of diseases]." These statements are, however, only beliefs. They are based on the limitations of modern medical science, a highly scientific and technologically advanced approach to the treatment of disease, and they are delivered to the patient by a highly educated individual in a society that defers to expertise. These pronouncements, which are in some cases death sentences, are quickly accepted by most patients and become a part of their own belief system. The vast majority of people with terminal diseases who accept whatever their doctors tell them (these patients are called "compliant") die very close to their predicted life-expectancy. By contrast, patients who challenge their physician's "death sentence" tend to survive much longer, and some of them go on to achieve full recoveries. In *Love, Medicine, and Miracles*, Bernie Siegel, M.D., vividly describes how the beliefs and attitudes of many of his cancer patients affected the outcome of their disease.

Most of the beliefs held by Americans have been defined by the standards, or norms, of our society, but how well does the norm fit you, a unique individual? If all of us attempted to conform, the world would be a boring place, devoid of creativity and innovation. We certainly wouldn't be enjoying the ease of living that technology has provided us were it not for the adventurous few who deviated from the conventional belief system.

Unfortunately, in every culture there is great pressure to conform. It isn't easy, to say the least, to hold beliefs that run counter to prevalent attitudes. Society, friends, and family all tell us we have strayed with phrases such as "You should . . . ," "You ought to . . . ," or—if your belief has caused them a lot of discomfort—"You're crazy!" Most of the time we respond to this pressure by giving up our unreasonable, or even outrageous, beliefs. Ultimately almost all of us would prefer to be accepted and loved by others; besides, we tell ourselves, "It wasn't that big a deal anyway."

Your belief system has a profound impact on your life: what you eat and think; how you dress and behave; what you do for a living; who you choose to marry, befriend, or live with; how you spend your leisure time; what your values and goals are; and how you define health and quality of life. It also determines the nature of the silent messages you give yourself every day. All of us talk to ourselves, and this internal dialog has a great deal to do with our state of mental health. These messages may be generally self-critical ("You stupid . . ." "Why did I say that?" "Why did I do that?" "How could I . . . ?" "I should've [could've] . . ."); limiting ("I'll never be able to . . ."); or accepting and supportive ("Good job!" "That's fine." "I did the best I could."). Almost all of my patients are very hard on themselves. They are self-critical and put themselves under a great deal of unnecessary pressure, while at the same time most are high achievers. As human beings we are imperfect; all of us make mistakes. The way we respond to these failings is what creates more, or lessens, stress in our lives. Our pattern of response is one we probably have been repeating reflexively since childhood.

A very simple yet powerful exercise that can help you become more conscious of your thoughts, beliefs, and emotions is to devote fifteen minutes writing out all that you are thinking during that time. Do this when you are not likely to be disturbed and don't edit anything out. After a few days of practicing this technique, many of your predominant beliefs will have been expressed on paper. Read them over. If they don't feel nurturing, build confidence and self-esteem, or regenerate you, clearly they are not serving you and need to be either eliminated or changed. Pay particular attention to the *should's*, *could's*, and *never's*. Before you discard what you write, examine your statements for possible clues to aspects of your life that may require more of your attention. For instance, if one of your statements reads, "I hate going to work," more than likely you may need to change your attitude about your job, or leave it for one that is more fulfilling and better suited to your talents. (If the thought of leaving your job raises the thought "How will I provide for myself and my family?" realize that this in itself can be a limiting thought. Numerous options will become available to you once you liberate yourself from your old assumptions and beliefs.)

Once you have identified beliefs that are holding you back from your goals and desires, or negatively impacting your health, the next step is to begin to *reprogram* your mind with thoughts, ideas, and images more aligned to what you want. One of the most effective ways to do this is through the use of **affirmations,** or positive thoughts that you repeat to yourself either verbally or in writing in order to produce a specific outcome. Affirmations are positive statements repeated frequently, always in the present tense, containing only positive words, and serve as a response to an often-heard negative message or as expression of a goal. For example, if some of the previous critical messages sound familiar to you, two affirmations that would help counteract them are "I love and approve of myself" and "I am always doing the best I can." These positive thoughts create images that directly affect the unconscious, shaping patterns of thought to direct behavior. In doing so, they act as powerful tools to unleash and stimulate the healing energy of love present in great abundance within each of us.

The purpose of affirmations is to replace habitual, limiting thought patterns and beliefs with more nurturing images of how you want your life to be. When affirmations are practiced regularly, they have the power to create optimal health by infusing the immune system with the life energy of *hope,* which triggers the activity of neuropeptides in the cells. Affirmations can be used to address virtually all aspects of your life, enhancing self-esteem, improving the quality of relationships, dealing with illness, and launching a more rewarding career.

Because of the simple nature of affirmations, the greatest challenge in using them is to suspend judgment long enough to allow them to produce the results you desire. When people begin repeating affirmations, they usually don't believe what they're saying (that's why they're saying them), although they would like to. Using affirmations is like reprogramming a computer. Your subconscious mind is the computer that has been receiving the same message for years—as the direct result of the thoughts and beliefs you have held for most, if not all, of your life. Now you are going to change the input with new "software."

Most computers have a total capacity for processing information far beyond the ability of the majority of computer operators to access it. Similarly, neuroscientists believe that the average person uses only 5 to 10 percent of his or her total brain capacity. As mentioned earlier, this average person has about fifty thousand thoughts every day, and it is estimated that 95 percent of them are the same ones he or she had the day before. Since your brain is hearing the same "program" repeated over and over again, it's no wonder you are able to realize only a small fraction of your (and your brain's) full potential. *Mental health will help to develop your creativity—you'll be recreating yourself—while allowing yourself greater access to the parts of your brain that have been dormant. It is in that recreational process that you'll find an almost limitless supply of joy and passion, along with some strong doses of pain to keep you on track.*

The best time to say your affirmation is immediately following the negative message you repeatedly give yourself. When you're feeling the frustration of recurring joint pain and thinking to yourself "This will never go away," you can follow that hopeless comment with the affirmation: "My knees [hip, back, shoulder] are healing and getting stronger every day." Positive statements like this while you're in the midst of changing your diet, taking the supplements, and following the rest of the Arthritis Survival Program will not only help to feel a little better but will also increase your level of hope. And as your arthritis improves, you'll believe the affirmation more and more until it is actually true.

Louise L. Hay has written a wonderful book on self-healing called *You Can Heal Your Life,* in which she focuses on the healing potential of affirmations as a means of learning to love yourself. Her book contains a list of medical conditions, each with the probable emotional cause and a corresponding affirmation. The emotional issues that she believes are most often associated with arthritis are *feeling unloved, criticism,* and *resentment.* The affirmation she recommends is: "I am love. I now choose to love and approve of myself. I see others with love." In her book *Anatomy of the Spirit,* Caroline Myss also mentions the mental and emotional issues associated with arthritis as *low self-esteem, self-confidence,* and *self-respect; sensitivity to criticism; fear and intimidation*; and *lack of trust.* Although these issues may not relate to you, I have used both books as references for many years and have found them to be consistently accurate. Think about how this information relates to you while also considering the content of your often-heard silent messages. If you find that one or more of these specific issues applies to you, then I would recommend creating affirmations to help lessen the harmful impact they may be having on your joints.

There are a variety of ways to use affirmations. Some people find they get their best results by writing each affirmation ten to twenty times a day. Others prefer to say them out loud, or to record them onto a cassette that they can then play to themselves daily. One powerful technique suggested by Louise Hay is to stare into a mirror and make eye contact with your reflection while verbally repeating each affirmation. Hay notes that this experience tends to bring up feelings of discomfort at first, and recommends that you continue the process until such feelings lessen or fade away altogether. You can experiment with these and other methods until you find the one that works best for you. Here are some other guidelines to insure that you get the best results from your affirmation program:

(1) **Always state your affirmation in the present tense and keep it positive.** For example, if one of your goals is to be free of job-related stress, the affirmation *I accomplish my daily responsibilities with ease and satisfaction* will produce far more effective results than statements such as *My job no longer makes me stressful.* The reason affirmations work is because the unconscious accepts them as statements of fact, and immediately begins to reorganize your life experience to match what you are telling it. So state *what you*

desire, not what you wish to be free from, and write and say your affirmation in the present tense *as if your desire is already accomplished.*

(2) **Keep your affirmations short and simple, and no longer than two brief sentences.**

(3) **Say or write each affirmation at least ten to twenty times each day.**

(4) **Whenever you experience yourself thinking or hearing a habitual negative message, counteract it by focusing on your affirmation.** Over time, you will find that your tendency to give yourself negative messages will diminish.

(5) **Schedule a time each day to do your affirmations, and adhere to it.** Doing something regularly at the same time each day adds to the momentum of what you are trying to achieve, and eventually will become a positive, effortless habit.

(6) **Repeat your affirmations in the first, second, and third person, using your name in each variation.** Using affirmations in the first person addresses the mental conditioning you have given yourself, while affirmations in the second and third person help to release the conditioning you may have been accepting from others. For example, if your name is Tom and one of your goals is to make more money, you might write: *I, Tom, am earning enough money to satisfy all my needs and desires. You, Tom, are earning enough money to satisfy all your needs and desires. He, Tom, is earning enough money to satisfy all his needs and desires.* In each case, write out or repeat the affirmation ten times.

(7) **Make a commitment to practice your affirmations for at least sixty days or until you begin experiencing the result you desire.**

You can use affirmations to help change any belief that doesn't feel good to you, to help you achieve any goal, or to create the life of your dreams. Most of my patients have come in because of one or more chronic physical or mental problems. Their objectives are clear: to stop living with chronic pain, to stop having sinus infections, to get rid of allergies, to have more energy, to suffer less anxiety, and so forth. After they have begun to see a definite improvement in their physical condition, which is usually after they have been working on the physical and environmentmal aspects of the Sinus or Arthritis Survival Program for one to three months, I recommend that they create a "wish list" in the form of affirmations. The following is a powerful exercise for transforming your life and creating optimal mental health:

- **List your greatest talents and gifts.** You have several. These are things that are most special about you, or that you do better than most other people. Ask yourself, "What do I most appreciate about myself?"
- **Next, list the things you most enjoy**—both activities and states of being, for example, "I really enjoy just being in the mountains, or on a beach." There will be some overlap with your first list. Many of the activities you enjoy doing are the things you're best at.
- **Next, list the things that have the most meaning for you.** This is important, because if your goal doesn't meaningfully encompass more than one area of your life, or have benefit to others in some way, more than likely it is incomplete, and you will lack the passion necessary to commit to it. As you list the meaningful things in your life, you will more easily recognize the talents and activities you enjoy that are most worth your while.
- **Now make a wish list of all your goals or objectives in every realm of your life**—physical/environmental, mental, emotional, social, and spiritual. Physical and environmental goals can include recovering from illnesses or ailments, engaging in or mastering a particular physical activity (anything you've ever considered doing), or living or working in a certain place. Mental goals might address career plans, financial

objectives, and any limiting beliefs that you'd like to change. Emotional goals have to do with feelings and self-esteem. Social goals are about your relationships with other people, while spiritual objectives have to do with your relationship with God or Spirit. As you do this part of the exercise, ask yourself, "What does my ideal life look like?" "Where do I see myself five or ten years from now?" "What is my purpose—what am I here to do?" Do *not* give yourself a time frame within which to attain any of these goals, and remember, it is *not* necessary to have a plan for getting there.

- **Next, reword all of your goals into affirmations.** For example, a goal might be "I'd like to cure my arthritis." Some simple affirmations might be: "My knees, [hips, back, shoulder] are now completely healed" or "My knees are getting better every day." Then compile a list of about ten affirmations that address your most important goals and desires, and the most limiting beliefs or critical messages that you'd like to change.

  Many people with arthritis have low self-esteem and are handicapped (unable to move forward in life) by their fear of making mistakes, sensitivity to criticism, and lack of trust. An extremely valuable affirmation for arthritis might be *"I'm always doing the best I can. There are no mistakes only lessons."*

- **Recite this entire list at least once a day, and whenever you hear a negative, limiting, or critical message, recite the one affirmation that corresponds to that message.** Or you can record them onto a cassette and listen to them in your own voice. Perhaps the most effective method for deriving benefit from affirmations is to *write, recite,* and *visualize* them (see "Guided Imagery and Visualization" below). Using this method, you would write down your affirmation while reciting it aloud, and then close your eyes and imagine what the affirmation looks and/or feels like, engaging as many of your senses as possible. If you can't picture it, it helps to *feel* your affirmations as you recite or write them, since this brings more energy to the experience. Make the process as vivid and real as possible.

I learned this technique from a patient, a man who owns an oil company and works part-time as a psychotherapist. He'd had a terrible case of chronic sinusitis for many years. On our second session, one month into the Sinus Survival Program, I presented this idea of changing some of his limiting, critical, or negative beliefs and clarifying his goals and objectives as a foundation of greater mental health. Shortly after this visit, he formulated a lengthy list of affirmations and goals. Once each day he recited every one of his new beliefs, then wrote them down on a sheet of paper, and after each one he closed his eyes and visualized what that desire or goal would look or feel like. When I next saw him, just over two months later, he told me that he had been repeating this procedure of reciting, writing, and visualizing for sixty consecutive days. He was thrilled to report to me that at least half of his affirmations and goals had already become a reality, including healthy sinuses! He continues to practice this method (using new affirmations) along with the physical and environmental health recommendations that he had implemented at the outset of the program. It is now more than seven years since my third session with him. During that time he has had only two sinus infections, and his chronic sinusitis remains cured.

My patients' affirmation/goal lists provide a blueprint of our work together. The lists also become their personal vision and give direction to their own self-healing process.

You must be able to clarify your desires to have any chance of obtaining them, and as you do this exercise, try to be as specific as possible. The next step is to believe, however minimally, that it is possible for you to meet these goals. The more you repeat the affirmations, the stronger your belief will become.

The third step in this formula for self-realization is *expectation*. The stronger your belief and the more objectives you have already reached, the higher will be your level of expectation. After my chronic sinusitis was cured, I developed the belief that anything is possible, a belief that has helped me to realize other dreams. Whatever it is that you *desire,* as long as you *believe* it's possible, you can *expect* it to happen. It is not necessary to know how, or to have a definite plan. Just be patient and flexible and be willing to accept the result, even if the "package" in which it arrives is different from what you had envisioned. If your objectives are clear, your intuition will help you make the right decisions to get what you want. Remember that you can always choose what to believe. Rather than continuing with the attitude "I'll believe it when I see it," why not try "When I believe it, then I'll see it."

I've repeatedly seen this technique change lives in a variety of ways other than disease. My favorite example is a woman from Tennessee whom I was treating for chronic fatigue, allergies, and sinusitis. In the early years of my holistic practice, I worked with a number of patients long-distance over the phone, never actually meeting them in person. An RN in her fifties, she taught in a nursing school in a small town and had never married, although she wanted to. She had resisted putting marriage on her goal list because, as she explained to me, "I know all the eligible men in town and in my church, and there aren't any possible candidates." I convinced her to include it on her goal list, and her affirmation read simply: *I am happily married.* Within a few months, she received a letter from a former professor of hers with whom she had a friendship years earlier. His wife had died the year before, and he wanted to visit his former student. Within months they were engaged, and a year after beginning her affirmation she was happily married. Her tears of joy over the phone and her gratitude left me in tears as well. We both felt as if we had experienced a miracle.

How you choose to see your arthritis or any other chronic condition can play a vital role in the way the disease affects you and whether or not it goes away. Some of the early reactions to a chronic or life-threatening disease are denial ("There must be some mistake"), anger and frustration ("Why me?" "What terrible luck"), self-pity ("I'll never be able to enjoy life again"), and resignation ("I'll just have to put up with it and continue to live this way for the rest of my life"). All of these are quite normal and understandable responses to something as devastating as an incurable condition. However, if you are interested in healing yourself, it is important to get beyond this point and look at your disease in a different light. According to Bernie Siegel, who contributed the following material to the book *Chop Wood, Carry Water,* you have several choices:

- **Accept your illness.** Being resigned to an illness can be destructive and can allow the illness to run your life, but accepting it allows energy to be freed for other things in your life.
- **See the illness as a source of growth.** If you begin to grow psychologically in response to the loss the illness has created in your life, then you don't need to have a physical illness anymore.
- **View your illness as a positive redirection in your life.** This means that you don't have to judge anything that happens to you. If you get fired from a job, for example, assume that you are being redirected toward something else you are supposed to be doing. Your entire life changes when you say that something is just a redirection. You are then at peace. Everything is okay and you go on your way, knowing that the new direction is the one that is intrinsically right for you. After a while you begin to *feel* that this is true.
- **Death or recurrence of illness is no longer seen as synonymous with failure after the aforementioned steps are accomplished, but simply as further choices or steps.** If staying alive were your sole goal, you would have to be a failure because you do have to die someday. However, when you begin to accept the inevitability of death and see that you have only a limited time, you begin to realize that you might as well enjoy the present to the best of your ability.
- **Learn self-love and peace of mind, and the body responds.** Your body gets "live" or "energy" messages when you say "I love myself." That's not the ego talking, it's self-esteem. It's as if someone else is loving you, saying that you are a worthwhile person, believing in you, and telling you that you are here to give something to the world. When you do that, your immune system says, "This person likes living; let's fight for his or her life."

- **Don't make physical change your sole goal.** Seek peace of mind, acceptance, and forgiveness. Learn to love. In the process, the disease won't be totally overlooked: It will be seen as one of the problems you are having, and perhaps one of your fears. If you learn about hope, love, acceptance, forgiveness, and peace of mind, the disease may go away in the process.
- **Achieve immortality through love.** The only way you can live forever is to love somebody. Then you can really leave a gift behind. When you live that way, as many people with physical illnesses do, it is even possible to decide when you die. You can say, "Thank you, I've used my body to its limit. I have loved as much as I possibly can, and I'm leaving at two o'clock today." And you go. Then maybe you have spent half an hour dying and the rest of your life living; but when these things are not done, you may spend a lot of your life dying, and only a little living.

I realize that most of you do not have a terminal disease, just a bad case of arthritis, but each of these options for looking at physical illness can work for you as a form of preventive medicine. In my experience, chronic pain and imminent death have provided the greatest motivation for people to change, but why wait until you have reached that point of crisis?

GUIDED IMAGERY AND VISUALIZATION

Visualization is a skill all of us have and one that we use every day. Most of the time, however, we do so unconsciously, such as when we daydream. The fifty thousand thoughts we have each and every day are often accompanied by inner pictures, or imagery, with corresponding emotions.

Since the 1970's, researchers, physicians, and other health care professionals have been examining how to harness these mental images in order to use them consciously to create improved states of well-being. Due to their continued work, thousands of

individuals nationwide are learning how to use visualization and guided imagery to enhance their health. In many cases their results have been astounding. Since 1971, radiation oncologist O. Carl Simonton, M.D., for instance, has been a pioneer in developing imagery as a self-care tool for cancer patients to use to bolster their response rate to traditional cancer treatments, with remarkable success. The first patient to whom he taught his techniques was a 61-year-old man who had been diagnosed with a "hopeless" case of throat cancer. In conjunction with his radiation treatments, the man spent five to fifteen minutes three times a day imagining himself healthy. Within two months he was completely cancer-free.

A similarly remarkable case is that of Garrett Porter, a patient of Patricia Norris, Ph.D., another leader in the field of guided imagery. Garrett was 9 and had been diagnosed with an inoperable brain tumor. Using biofeedback techniques in conjunction with imagery based on Garrett's favorite TV show, *Star Trek* (he pictured missiles striking and destroying his tumor), Garrett was able to completely reverse his condition within a year, with brain scans confirming his tumor's disappearance.

Numerous studies also confirm the health benefits of imagery and visualization. For example, college volunteers who practiced imagery twice daily for six weeks experienced a marked increase in salivary immunoglobulin A as compared to a control group who did not practice imagery. In another study, the well-known drop in helper T immune cells in students facing the stress of final examinations was greatly reduced in a group utilizing relaxation and imagery each day for a month before exams. And patients scheduled for gall bladder surgery who listened to imagery tapes before and after their operations had less wound inflammation, lower cortisone levels, and less anxiety than did controls who were treated with comparable periods of quiet only.

Like most of the other therapies outlined in this chapter, one of the most exciting things about guided imagery and visualization is that both techniques are powerful self-healing tools that can be used to create positive change in almost any area of your life. Besides physical health, imagery can help you feel more peaceful and relaxed, assist you in further developing your creative talents, create more fulfillment in your relationships, improve your ability to achieve career goals, and dissolve negative habit patterns. All that is necessary is a commitment to practice the techniques on a regular basis.

Guided imagery and visualization work to improve and maintain health because of their ability to directly affect our bodies at a cellular level, particularly with regard to neuropeptides. In addition, the use of imagery can often provide greater insight into causes and treatment for chronic conditions, guiding us toward the most personalized and effective solutions for our particular health problems. This occurs because our mental images are so deeply connected to our emotions, which, as we have discussed, are usually interconnected with the events in our lives. By using imagery, you can become better aware of what emotional issues may lie beneath the surface of your life and begin the process of healing them.

There are two types of guided imagery and visualization: preconceived or preselected images employed by you or your health care professional in order to address a specific problem and achieve a specific outcome, such as healing an arthritic joint; and imagery that occurs spontaneously as you sit comfortably, eyes closed and breathing freely. Both forms have value, so try them both and see which works best for you. What follows are two techniques you can use to make imagery a part of your Arthritis Survival Program. The first is a form of guided imagery, while the latter is conducive for allowing spontaneous imagery to occur on its own.

The Remembrance Technique. This exercise can be adapted to improve issues or conditions in any area of your life. It's called the Remembrance Technique because in our core selves we are already whole. In many respects, healing is simply a remembrance of that state in order to reconnect with it. Begin this exercise by sitting comfortably in a chair or lying down in bed. Select a time and place when you will not be disturbed. Close your eyes and focus on your breathing. Take a few deep, unforced breaths to help you relax. With each inhalation, imagine that soothing, relaxing energy is flowing through all areas of your body. As you exhale, visualize the cares and concerns of the day gradually disappearing. Do this for two or three minutes, allowing your breath to carry you to a place of calm relaxation.

Now choose the issue you want to focus on for the rest of the exercise, and recall a time when the outcome you desire was something you have already experienced. For example, if you have hip pain, remember a time when you were in excellent health and could move freely without pain. Allow yourself to re-experience that time, using all of your senses to make what you are imagining as vivid as possible. Once you have reconnected to the experience, bring it into the present *as if it were actually happening now.* Stay with the experience for at least five more minutes, mentally affirming that you *are* experiencing the state you desire here in the present.

Another form of preselected imagery is to focus on an image of a healthy joint: a perfectly smooth, slippery, white, glistening, radiant cartilage covering the surfaces of the arthritic knee, hip, spine, or shoulder that has been causing you so much pain. Prepare yourself in the same way I've described above: sitting, relaxed, and focused on breath. Even though this is a preselected image (like Garrett Porter's missiles striking his tumor), it can also be a dynamic process in which the image changes and evolves with each session of imagery. You might envision masons patching defects or holes in the surface of the degenerative cartilage with a "cement" that resembles healthy cartilage during one imagery session. Another time, you might see a radiant white light filling every cartilaginous cell and restoring it to perfect health with every inhalation you take, and on exhalation the toxins and mineral debris within the cartilage are expelled and disintegrate. Allow your imagery to be creative without placing any restrictions upon it. There is no one correct image to use for healing arthritis. Whatever works for you and feels good is the "right" image.

Spontaneous imagery. In this exercise, instead of preselecting a specific outcome, you are going to allow your own unconscious to communicate with you through imagery about whatever situation in your life you choose to focus on. As in the preceding exercise, sit or lie down comfortably in a quiet place, close your eyes, and focus on your breath until you feel yourself settling into a deeper state of relaxation. Now focus on the physical problem you'd like to heal or the area in your life into which you desire to gain greater insight, allowing thoughts and images to freely and spontaneously emerge. Although you may have chosen your arthritic joint to focus on, you may be surprised by what you experience, but don't judge it. Trust that your unconscious knows what you most need to understand, and allow your imagery to lead you to that answer. Continue this exercise for five to ten minutes, and when you complete it, write down what you experienced so that you can contemplate it for possible further insight. As a variation to this exercise, you can first ask a question of yourself, such as "Why do I have arthritis?" or "What do I have to learn from my arthritis?" and then see what image appears. From there, you may find yourself engaged in a dialog between yourself and your unconscious that results in answers and solutions you did not know were possible.

When you first begin to practice mental imagery techniques, don't be discouraged if at first "nothing seems to be happening." Like any new skill, achieving results in imagery takes time. Remember that the language of your unconscious, like the symbolism of your dreams, is usually not literal or rational. It may take some time before you are able to grasp the messages of the images you perceive. Keeping a written log of your experience can make learning this new "language" easier.

OPTIMISM AND HUMOR

In the Bible it is written: "A cheerful heart is good medicine, but a downcast spirit dries up the bones" (Proverbs 17:22). Science is now beginning to verify this ancient truth, revealing that optimism and humor are integral factors in one's overall health, providing both physical and mental benefits. One of the most famous anecdotes illustrating this point concerns Norman Cousins, who, in his book *Anatomy of an Illness*, attributed his recovery from ankylosing spondylitis (a potentially crippling arthritic condition of the spine) to the many hours he spent watching Marx Brothers movies and reruns of *Candid Camera* while taking megadoses of vitamin C. The more he laughed, the more his pain diminished, until eventually his illness completely disappeared, never to return. Based on his experience with humor, Cousins went on to explore mind/body medicine at UCLA. Today a number of institutions are studying the healing potential of humor, such as the appropriately named Gesundheit Institute in Arlington, Virginia, founded and directed by Patch Adams, M.D.

Some of the most in-depth research in this area has been conducted by Robert Ornstein, Ph.D., and David Sobel, M.D., who presented their findings in their book *Healthy Pleasures.* They discovered that the people who are optimally healthy also tend to be optimistic and happy, and possess the belief that things will work out no matter what their difficulties may be. Such people maintain a vital sense of humor about life and enjoy a good laugh, often at their own expense. According to Ornstein and Sobel, they also expect good things of life, including being liked and respected by others, and experience pleasure in most of what they do. They usually look at stressful situations as temporary setbacks, specific to the immediate circumstance and due largely to external causes. Pessimists, on the other hand, when faced with life-challenging events, tend to think they will be permanent ("It's going to last forever"), generalize the problems to their whole lives ("It's going to spoil everything"), and blame themselves ("It's my fault"). Recent research at the Mayo Clinic suggests that pessimism is a significant risk factor for early death. Over eight hundred patients were given a personality test that categorized them as optimistic, mixed, or pessimistic. After their health status was evaluated thirty years later, the pessimists had a significantly higher-than-expected death rate.

Optimistic people also tend to laugh a lot, something that

most likely plays an important role in their health. Studies have shown that laughter can strengthen the immune system. One study, for instance, found that test subjects who watched video-tapes of the comedian Richard Pryor produced increased levels of antibodies in their saliva. Furthermore, subjects in the study who said they frequently used humor to cope with life stress had consistently higher baseline levels of those antibodies that help to combat infections such as colds.

Hearty laughter is actually a form of gentle exercise, or "inner jogging." Describing the physiological effects of laughter, Ornstein and Sobel write:

> A robust laugh gives the muscles of your face, shoulders, diaphragm, and abdomen a good workout. With convulsive or side-splitting laughter, even your arm and leg muscles come into play. Your heart rate and blood pressure temporarily rise, breathing becomes faster and deeper, and oxygen surges through your bloodstream. A vigorous laugh can burn up as many calories per hour as brisk walking or cycling.
>
> The afterglow of a hearty laugh is positively relaxing. Blood pressure may temporarily fall, your muscles go limp, and you bask in a mild euphoria. Some researchers speculate that laughter triggers the release of endorphins, the brain's own opiates; this may account for the pain relief and euphoria that accompany laughter.

In short, laughter's benefits are many and profound. Unfortunately most of us don't laugh enough. One recent study found that young children laugh about 400 times a day, while the average adult laughs only 14 times. When the question posed to octogenarians is "If you had your life to live over again, what would you do differently?" the answer often is "I'd take life much less seriously." Comedian George Burns, who lived to 100, wrote the book *Wisdom of the 90's* at age 95. He attributed his ability to laugh at himself as well as loving what he did for a living as the most important factors in his longevity.

Both optimism and a sense of humor are directly related to

our beliefs. If you wish to become more optimistic and experience more humor and fun in your life, practice the exercises outlined in this chapter. It may take time before you achieve the results you desire, but your commitment will prove well worth it and will impact your mood, mental health, and even survival. Nothing quite epitomizes the free flow of life force energy as laughter, and all of us can stand to laugh even more than we do. Be advised, however. There is one side effect to this powerful form of self-healing: more pleasure.

EMOTIONAL HEALTH

The emotionally fit are able to identify their feelings and can express, fully experience, and accept them as well. I have heard contemporary American culture referred to as the "no-feeling" society. The feelings are certainly present, but as a result of our lifestyle we have constructed such formidable protective barriers around ourselves that to a great extent we have become unconscious of our feelings, especially the more uncomfortable ones.

There are those who believe there are only two basic human emotions: love and fear. The so-called negative or painful emotions, such as anger, grief, anxiety, depression, envy, guilt, hatred, hostility, jealousy, loneliness, shame, and worry, are all expressions of fear. The feelings of acceptance, intimacy, joy, power, approval, and peacefulness are all aspects of love. The greater our degree of fear, the less capable we are of experiencing love.

With any chronic illness, including arthritis, fear becomes the predominant emotion. When this occurs, your greatest liability is your *loss of love*—for yourself and those closest to you. It becomes a much greater challenge to nurture yourself and to feel fully alive when you're consumed with the anxiety and insecurity created by your ongoing physical discomfort and disability. You may also be frequently hearing the silent messages "This is only going to get worse" or "I'm going to have to live this way for the rest of my life." When someone develops moderate to severe arthritis, they experience a significant loss of physical mobility along with a diminished enjoyment of life. Many people derive a great deal of their self-esteem, self-confidence, and self-respect from their physical mobility and their ability to perform well physically (even the most basic tasks). If their disability is great enough, it may also impair their capacity to care for themselves or a loved one, which further diminishes self-esteem. As a result, a deep sadness and depression often accompany fear in people with arthritis.

Some mental health professionals consider four basic emotions: love or joy, sadness, anger, and fear. So at any given moment you're feeling either glad, sad, mad, or scared, or some combination of these. In our culture it is not socially acceptable to express most of the "negative" emotions, and men especially are not supposed to show signs of weakness or insecurity or to cry ("Big boys don't cry"). The majority of us have learned to repress these feelings until we are unaware that we even have them. Society has helped us suppress our painful (negative) feelings by perpetuating the myth of an emotionally pain-free existence. The numerous ads in the media for analgesics to treat the pain of arthritis and headaches, and the common use of alcohol or drugs to dull the pain of an awkward social situation or personal crisis, give us the clear message that *not only is pain a bad thing, but life can be pain free.*

If we spend less time avoiding emotional pain, but instead focus our attention on it, accept it, and relax into it, the pain will diminish or even disappear. *If we continue to ignore and repress it, it often manifests itself as physical pain, illness, or disease.* Redford Williams, M.D., a researcher in behavioral medicine at the Duke University Medical Center, has gathered a wealth of data suggesting that chronic anger is so damaging to the body that it ranks with, or even exceeds, cigarette smoking, obesity, and a high-fat diet as a powerful risk factor for early death. Williams reported that people who scored high on a hostility scale as teenagers were much more likely than their more cheerful peers to have elevated cholesterol levels as adults, suggesting a link between unremitting anger and heart disease.

In another study, Dr. Mara Julius, an epidemiologist at the

University of Michigan, analyzed the effects of chronic anger on women over a period of eighteen years. She found that women who had answered initial test questions with obvious signs of long-term, suppressed anger were three times more likely to have *died* during the study than those women who did not harbor such hostile feelings. Chronic sinusitis is usually associated with a tremendous amount of unexpressed anger, and I've also found it to be the primary trigger for most colds and sinus infections, as well as being an important contributing factor to arthritis and many other chronic conditions.

Clyde Reid is director of the Center for New Beginnings in Denver. In his insightful book *Celebrate the Temporary,* he says, "Leaning into life's pain can also be a lifestyle, and is far more satisfying than the avoidance style. It requires small doses of plain courage to look pain in the eye, but it prepares you for more serious pain when it comes. In the meantime, all the energy expended to avoid pain is now available for the business of living."

I am not advocating that you seek out painful experiences, nor am I proposing that you endure prolonged or persistent pain. That is called suffering. Health and happiness do not have prerequisites that require you to suffer. Life is to be enjoyed, but the notion that it can be lived entirely without painful feelings is an unhealthy belief. Pain and joy are intertwined, and **the more you allow yourself to accept, embrace, and feel both pain and joy, the greater will be your sense of emotional health.**

Of the mental-emotional connection, Albert Ellis, a psychologist and founder of the Institute for Rational-Emotive Therapy in New York City, has said that "virtually all 'emotionally disturbed' individuals actually think crookedly, magically, dogmatically, and unrealistically." David D. Burns, M.D., a psychiatrist and author of *The Feeling Good Handbook* writes:

> Certain kinds of negative thoughts make people unhappy. In fact, I believe that unhealthy, negative emotions—depression, anxiety, excessive anger, inappropriate guilt, etc.—are *always* caused

by illogical, distorted thoughts, even if those thoughts may seem absolutely valid at the time. By learning to look at things more realistically, by getting rid of your distorted thinking patterns, you can break out of a bad mood, often in a short period of time, without having to rely on medication or prolonged psychotherapy.

Burns offers the following list of thought distortions:

- **All-or-nothing thinking.** You classify things into absolute, black-and-white categories.
- **Overgeneralization.** You view a single negative situation as a never-ending pattern of defeat.
- **Mental filtering.** You dwell on negatives and overlook positives.
- **Discounting the positive.** You insist your accomplishments or positive qualities "don't count."
- **Magnification or minimization.** You blow things out of proportion or shrink their importance inappropriately.
- **Making *should* statements.** You criticize yourself and others by using the terms *should, shouldn't, must, ought,* and *have to.*
- **Emotional reasoning.** You reason from how you feel. If you feel like an idiot, you assume you must be one. If you don't feel like doing something, you put it off.
- **Jumping to conclusions.** You "mind-read," assuming, without definite evidence of it, that people are reacting negatively to you. Or you "fortune-tell," arbitrarily predicting bad outcomes.
- **Labeling.** You identify with your shortcomings. Instead of saying, "I made a mistake," you tell yourself, "I'm such a jerk . . . a real loser."
- **Personalization and blame.** You blame yourself for something you weren't entirely responsible for, or you blame others and ignore the impact of your own attitudes or behavior.

As I've already said, negative thoughts and the feelings they engender contribute to physical illness. The low self-esteem and sensitivity to criticism found in many people with arthritis are frequently associated with several of the above thought distortions. These repeated thoughts will often trigger anger (ultimately with ourselves) and depression (almost always fueled by repressed anger), which, if not expressed, can further diminish self-esteem and aggravate arthritic pain. Many of these same critical and limiting messages are also preventing you from achieving your goals and seeing your "wish list" become a reality. These theories of Drs. Ellis and Burns constitute the foundation of cognitive psychotherapy—the form of counseling I've found to be highly effective for my patients.

One self-care approach you might try for gaining greater self-awareness is to attempt to identify the mental and emotional issues that may have contributed to causing your arthritis. A method I've used with my patients for many years is to consider the possible benefits or secondary gain resulting from having this condition. They may not be readily apparent, but if you're open to this introspective exploration, you'll usually find some answers, however minimal, to the question "What are the benefits of having arthritis?" They may include "I don't have to work as hard [or at all]"; "I can collect disability"; "I was able to take early retirement"; "My husband [or wife] pays more attention to me and, to a much greater extent, now has to take care of me"; "I'm no longer expected to perform at the level I had been, and that has reduced a lot of pressure [stress] that I'd been feeling." Whether it's more attention, a need to be cared for, job dissatisfaction, performance anxiety, or some other unmet need, I believe there are almost always some secondary gains associated with every chronic disease. Since you did not respond preventively, in order to meet those unconscious needs, your body created an illness. If these not-so-subtle benefits can be understood and you become more aware of what your needs and desires are, it will help considerably in identifying the emotional causes of your physical problem and allow you to work on resolving them. Once you have become aware of the issues, you can then begin expressing your emotions while addressing the unmet needs your feelings have revealed. The process continues with acceptance: knowing that it's okay to feel whatever you're feeling. This healing process will not only lead you to emotional health, it will help you practice preventive medicine, and will also take you a giant step closer to being free of your degenerative joint dis-ease. Remember, a basic tenet of mind-body medicine is that *your core issues are held in your tissues.*

BREATHWORK AND MEDITATION

The benefits of learning to breathe properly and consciously go far beyond the physical. Proper breathing can also improve your mood, make you mentally more alert, and help you to become more aware of deeply held and often painful feelings. Most importantly, by working with your breathing, you can begin to heal the wounded, rejected, unacknowledged, and disowned parts of yourself and bring them into wholeness.

The primary reason so many of us breathe unconsciously and inefficiently lies in the fact that our breathing process began traumatically at birth. We were forcibly expelled from the security of the womb and compelled to take our first breath on our own when we encountered the outside world. Often that first breath came as a harsh and unexpected shock, accompanied by pain and confusion. In order to suppress such pain, newborns typically follow their first inhalation by pausing and holding their breath for a moment as they struggle to make sense of their new environment. Today a number of researchers in the field of mental health speculate that this first pause in our breath not only sets the stage for a lifetime of shallow, inefficient breathing but also conditions us to suppress our painful emotions instead of learning how to accept and relax into them. You can observe this pattern in yourself the next time you find yourself feeling shock, fear, pain, or worry. If you take a moment to observe yourself in the initial experience of such emotions, more than likely you will find that you are also holding your breath or breathing very shallowly.

Breathwork, also known as "breath therapy," is a means of

learning how to breathe consciously and fully in order to deal with emotional pain more effectively and healthfully. There are many approaches to breathwork, ranging from ancient breathing techniques found in the traditions of *yoga, tai chi,* and *qigong,* to modern-day methods such as *rebirthing* (also known as *conscious connected breathing*), developed by Leonard Orr, and *holotropic breathwork,* developed by Stanislav Grof. All of them have in common a focus on the breath and the ability to move energy through the body and connect you with suppressed emotions and limiting beliefs in order to heal them.

Most breathwork therapies use the technique of connected breathing, first pioneered by Leonard Orr. In connected breathing, each inhalation immediately follows the exhalation of the preceding breath without pause. (Typically we breathe unconsciously, pausing between inhalation and exhalation.) The pattern of respiration can vary according to technique. Sometimes it is rapid; sometimes it is deep, slow, and full. In addition, some approaches recommend breathing in and out through the mouth, instead of the nose, and both abdominal and chest breathing can be used. In rebirthing, sometimes the therapy is performed in a tub or underwater with the use of a snorkel, although this usually does not occur until after the client has had a number of "dry" connected breathing sessions and has become comfortable with the movement of energy and integration of emotions that commonly occur during the rebirthing process. Because of the emotional release that can result from breathwork, it is advisable to learn the techniques under the direction of a skilled breath therapist. Once you gain proficiency, however, you will have at your disposal a powerful self-healing technique that you can practice daily on your own.

Meditation also offers a multitude of emotional health benefits. There are numerous meditation techniques, but all of them can be accurately described as conscious breathing methods. Meditation's many physiological benefits include improved immune function; reduced stress, including decreased levels of adrenaline, cortisone, and free radicals; increased oxygen intake; relief from chronic pain and headache; lower blood pressure and heart rate; and a reduction of core body temperature, which has been linked to increased longevity. Among the psychological benefits of meditation are greater relaxation; improved focus on the present instead of regrets and worries about the past and future; enhanced creativity and cognitive functioning; heightened spiritual awareness (including insights leading to the healing of past emotional trauma); improved awareness and management of beliefs and emotions; and a greater compassion and recognition of others and oneself as parts of a greater whole.

The following is a simple meditation technique that utilizes breathing to promote mental calm. Select a quiet place and sit in a chair with your back straight and your feet on the floor. Close your eyes and begin abdominal breathing, inhaling and exhaling through your nose at a rate of three to four full breaths (inhaled and exhaled) per minute. The object of this exercise is to stay focused on your breath, allowing whatever thoughts you have to come and go without being absorbed by them. Should you find your attention wandering, bring it back to your breath. You can also enhance the process by silently repeating a short affirmation, or a positive phrase, such as *God, love,* or *peace* on both the inhale and the exhale. At first, try to do this exercise for five minutes once or twice a day, gradually working up to twenty minutes twice daily. Don't be discouraged if at first you find this exercise difficult to practice. For most Americans, sitting and breathing without thinking or external stimulation is not easy. With time and continued practice, especially in the morning and before you go to bed, you will begin to notice the benefits meditation affords. (For more on meditation, see Chapter 6.)

DEALING WITH ANGER

Unexpressed anger, or anger that is expressed inappropriately, is both harmful and extremely common in our society. Most of us were taught very early in life that anger was an unacceptable emotion. When it was expressed, it often elicited fear in us, and was usually equated with bodily harm and loss of control ("He's really lost it"; "He's out of control"). This inability to safely express anger has been shown to produce many serious health consequences, from heart attacks to sinus infections. Today many psychotherapists are combining sound and body movement techniques to help their patients deal with their anger, finding that such approaches can be far more effective than simply talking about it. The following techniques can be safely employed by anyone to release the highly charged emotional energy of anger. They are most effective when employed regularly as preventive measures, instead of allowing anger to build up into a state of chronic, health-impacting tension, much less explosive rage.

Screaming. This is the most common anger release technique due to the fact that all of us already know how to do it. In his novel *Tai-Pan,* author James Clavell wrote that the chieftains of ancient Scotland for centuries maintained the custom of "the screaming tree." From the time they entered adolescence, males of the clan were instructed to go into the forest and select a tree to which they could express their discontent. Then, whenever their troubles grew too great to otherwise deal with, they would go to the forest alone and scream with the tree as their witness until their emotions settled.

The value of screaming is no secret to young children, who commonly scream when they are greatly upset, only to exhibit a smiling face moments afterward. For adults, the biggest difficulty involved is finding a place to scream in privacy. Screaming when you are home alone, in the basement or closet, in the car with the windows up, or in a secluded spot outside are all possibilities. To get the most benefit, take a deep abdominal breath before you scream, and then direct the scream from your diaphragm or deep within your chest cavity, as this will protect your vocal cords. As you scream, slowly move your upper body from side to side or up and down. Usually, after two or three screams in succession, you will begin to feel much better.

The angry letter (not sent). This technique is increasingly employed by therapists to help their clients release their anger. It involves writing a letter to the person with whom you are angry, listing all of the reasons why you are upset with them. As you write, allow yourself to express whatever comes to mind, no matter how harsh or offensive it may seem. Once the letter is written, read it over, and if anything else occurs to you that you wish to express, write that down, too, before signing it. Then either burn the letter or tear it up into small pieces.

Punching. Punching a bag, pillow, or sofa is another effective method of dissipating anger. Remember to grunt or yell with each punch. A variation of this method is to take hold of a pillow and hit it against the floor, sofa, or wall. With either approach, it takes only a few moments before you will start to feel your anger transforming into satisfaction and even joy. Remember, anger in and of itself is not a negative emotion to be shunned. It's only when it remains bottled up inside of us unexpressed that it becomes unhealthy. *Safely and appropriately expressing your anger in socially acceptable ways can dramatically improve the way you feel, both emotionally and physically.*

However, simply venting anger doesn't do the whole job. In fact, one study in April 1999 concluded that punching to release anger actually tends to increase and prolong feelings of hostility. Although this finding runs counter to my personal experience and that of many of my patients who have benefited from this practice, there are several additional steps that can be taken to release anger. You can start by recognizing that your anger may be the result of unreasonable or even irrational demands you've made on yourself or someone else, and that by maintaining these demands you are hurting yourself with increased stress. It is therefore in your best interest to release the demands and let go of the anger.

Aerobic exercise. This is another quick-fix method for dissipating anger and opening your nose and sinuses. However, if you're especially enraged about a particular incident or situation, wait at least twenty minutes and take some deep breaths before beginning a strenuous workout. There can be a greater risk of heart attack associated with exercise *immediately* following emotional trauma. Journaling, which I'll discuss in the next section, is also an effective means of releasing anger but not quite as fast as punching and exercise.

DREAMWORK AND JOURNALING

Dreams can play an important role in your healing journey. Serving as symbolic expressions of your inner emotional life, dreams often provide the clues you need to better understand your mental and emotional states, as well as the guidance you may need to heal personal life situations. Dreams can also sometimes reveal how to heal physical disease conditions. This was illustrated in a dream of Alexander the Great recounted in Pliny's *Natural History.* One of Alexander's friends, Ptolemaus, was dying of a poisoned wound, when Alexander dreamt of a dragon holding a plant in its mouth. The dragon said that the plant was the key to curing Ptolemaus. Upon awakening, Alexander dispatched soldiers to the place he had seen in his dream. They returned with the plant and, as the dream had predicted, Ptolemaus, as well as many others of Alexander's troops suffering from similar wounds, was cured.

In American society, dreams are often overlooked or ignored, although researchers like Stephen LaBarge, Ph.D., have in recent decades done much to scientifically demonstrate their importance. The two biggest obstacles that prevent us from getting the most benefit from our dreams are that we either do not remember or quickly forget them, or we do not know how to interpret the symbolism and imagery that dreams contain. Dream recall is a skill that anyone can develop with time and practice, however. One of the keys to dreamwork is to commit to focusing attention on your dreams. A deceptively simple way to do this is to tell yourself each night before you fall asleep that when you awaken you will remember what you dreamt during the night. At first you may not experience much success, but regular affirmation of this technique will instruct your unconscious to eventually make your dreams recallable.

As you start to remember your dreams, keep a pad and pencil or a tape recorder by your bed so that you can either write down or verbally record them immediately after you awaken. All of us dream an average of three or four times each night. With practice, many people who make the commitment to record and study their dreams are able to train themselves to spontaneously awaken after each dream cycle to record the gist of their dreams before settling back to sleep until after their next dream stage. Recording your dreams *immediately* after you awaken provides the best results, since dreams are quickly forgotten once you get out of bed and begin your day. Initially, all you may recall are fragments of your dream experience. Don't be discouraged if this is the case. Over time, the regular recording of your dreams will begin to yield more details. In addition, after you have recorded your dreams for a few weeks or months, as you read over your dream diary, you will start to notice how certain symbols and events tend to recur. Pay attention to such common themes: Usually they contain the most important messages that your dreams have for you.

Learning how to interpret the symbolism of your dreams takes time and practice. Certain psychotherapists, especially those with a background in Jungian theory, are skilled in dream interpretation and can help you, and a number of books on the subject can also guide you. Bear in mind, however, that your dreams are highly personal, and although many dream symbols do seem to be common to what Jung called "the collective unconscious," there is no such thing as a standard for dream interpretation that will work for everyone. As the dreamer of your own life, you are ultimately the person best suited to appreciate your dreams and discern their deepest meanings. By taking the time to do so, you can improve your mental and emotional health immeasurably.

Journaling is another simple but very effective way to become more conscious of your mental and emotional life and to help you better express your feelings. The practice of journaling entails keeping a written record of your thoughts, emotions, and any other daily experiences that you would like to better understand. Instead of recording your dreams, you will be keeping a journal of your waking activities. When journaling is done on a regular basis, it usually results in increased self-knowledge, often with insights that are both enlightening and enlivening. In a very real sense, journaling can help you become your own therapist or best friend: Instead of trying to express what you're feeling to someone else, through the process of journaling you tell it to yourself. The result is that your journal becomes your own emotional diary.

Many people who begin the practice of journaling are amazed to discover how the simple act of writing out one's daily experiences can lead to sudden or deeper insights into what they are feeling. Journaling can also help you become better aware of your beliefs, providing you with the opportunity to recognize and change those that may be limiting you. As you journal you will also start to take more control over what you are thinking and feeling, becoming less reactive to your life experiences and more creative in your approaches to dealing with them. Journaling also makes communicating with yourself easier and allows greater clarity, since you are free from judgment or criticism from others. Your journal is for you alone and isn't meant to be shared. Nor do you have to worry about spelling or grammar.

A number of researchers, including James W. Pennebaker, Ph.D., author of the book *Opening Up,* have documented the benefits that journaling can provide by writing about upsetting or traumatic experiences. For people who have difficulty expressing their emotions, particularly those that are judged to be negative, such as anger or fear, journaling can be especially valuable as a tool for self-healing. The results of a recent study measuring the effects of writing about stressful experiences on symptom reduction in patients with rheumatoid arthritis and asthma were published in *The Journal of the American Medical Association* in April 1999. The subjects in the study were asked to write about the most stressful event of their lives for twenty minutes for three consecutive days. They changed *nothing else* in their treatment regimen. Four months later, researchers found a significant reduction in the severity of disease in the arthritics and a marked improvement in lung function in the asthmatics.

For best results, try to write in your journal around the same time each day. This will help you make journaling a healthy habit. Just before you go to bed can be an ideal time for journaling. You can express the emotions that you've been containing all day and can provide resolution to the day's events prior to going to sleep. Journaling and dreamwork will not only help you to heal mentally and emotionally (and physically) but can also open up new vistas of adventure that can last you a lifetime.

WORK AND PLAY

Do you enjoy your job? Does your work utilize your greatest talents? Is your job fulfilling and challenging? Sadly, for the majority of Americans the answer to these questions is no. Recent studies reveal that an alarmingly high proportion of our society—nearly 70 percent of us—do not experience satisfaction from our jobs. Unfortunately, there is a significant price to be paid for not loving your work, both physiologically and psychologically. For example, in a study conducted by the Massachussetts Department of Health in the late 1980's, it was found that the two greatest risk factors for heart disease lie in one's self-happiness rating and one's level of job satisfaction. Low scores in these two areas were shown to be better indicators of the likelihood for developing heart disease than high cholesterol, high blood pressure, overweight, and a sedentary lifestyle. No wonder, then, that in the U.S. more heart attacks occur on Monday morning around nine o'clock than at any other time of the week.

Your job is a vital aspect of your mental health. If you find yourself working at a job that you do not enjoy, chances are that you continue to do so because of one or more of the following limiting beliefs: *I don't have a choice; I need the money; I'll never be able to make enough money doing what I love; I have no idea what I'd enjoy doing or what my greatest talents are.* By using the techniques outlined in this chapter, especially in the section "Beliefs, Attitudes, Goals, and Affirmations," you can begin to liberate yourself from these unhealthy beliefs. You'll discover that you are not bound to your job for life and you do have the ability to find a job for which you are better suited and that is more fulfilling. Every one of us is blessed with at least one God-given talent, and there is at least one activity that we enjoy doing that we do quite well. *That* is where you need to begin to investigate what your gifts are. Write down your talents as outlined in the goal-setting section above, followed by a list of activities you truly enjoy. Then brainstorm all the possible ways you can think of in which you can earn a living combining your talents with each of the activities you wrote down. List every idea that occurs to you, regardless of how ridiculous it may seem. As you continue to practice this exercise, you will have a much clearer idea of new job options. At the same time, acknowledge that you are seeking a greater level of fulfillment, are willing to change and take a risk, and are committed to begin the exploration that will lead you to work that you love doing. In the process, you may discover that your capabilities are limitless.

Even if you are fortunate to have a job you do enjoy, you may still be prey to another modern-day dis-ease, *workaholism.* According to the Economic Policy Institute in Washington, DC, the majority of Americans are working longer and harder than they used to. Our yearly workload has increased by 158 hours, compared to that of twenty years ago, including longer commuting times and less paid holidays and vacation time. That's the equivalent of an extra month's work per year. To counter this tendency, it is essential that you regularly engage in the counterbalance to work: *play.*

Many of us have unfortunately relegated play to childhood; yet, play is a crucial aspect of mental health and is unrivaled as a means of expressing joy, passion, exhilaration, even ecstasy. The word *play* comes from the Middle Dutch *pleyen,* which means "to dance, leap for joy, and rejoice," all activities that suggest a vibrantly healthy mental state. *Play* has also been defined as any activity in which you lose track of time. Believing that play is not appropriate adult behavior is both limiting and unhealthy.

If your work involves your greatest talents and is something you truly enjoy doing, work and play for you can seem virtually indistinguishable. Even so, to optimize mental health, find at least one other activity to participate in, besides your work, that you can thoroughly enjoy. Such activities include sports, games, dance, and active creative pursuits such as playing a musical instrument, acting, singing, painting, crafts, or gardening. Although many people derive great pleasure from playing cards, chess and other board games, or stamp or coin collecting, all of these are mental pursuits. To create a healthier balance, select activities that utilize your body, allow you to better express your feelings and creativity, and perhaps even bring you to a greater level of spiritual attunement. Ideally the activity should be something so consuming and absorbing that it requires your total attention, providing a pleasurable escape from your normal tension, stress, and habitual thought patterns. Choose something that instinctively appeals to you and do it on a regular basis, for at least an hour three times a week. Be prepared to make mistakes and look silly. That's part of the risk, and the excitement, of doing something new. The more you commit to and practice whatever activity you choose, the better you'll become at it and the more you'll enjoy the benefits it provides.

We live in a society where work has become the greatest addiction, and the majority of us gauge our self-worth according to our achievements and net worth. For this reason alone the importance of play cannot be overemphasized. All of us, for a short time at least, need to regularly let go of that responsible, mature, working adult part of ourselves to reconnect with our woefully neglected playful "inner child."

SUMMARY

The biggest obstacles each of us must overcome in order to achieve optimal mental and emotional health are our largely unconscious denial and repression of emotional pain, and our limiting thoughts, beliefs, and attitudes, which combined create our unhealthy behaviors. The tools in this chapter will enable you to heighten your awareness, allowing you to consciously transform your life in harmony with your greatest needs and desires. The more you practice the methods outlined here, the more profound the impact you will have on your mental health as well as your physical health and your arthritis. *You will become more conscious of your behavior and gain the freedom to choose how you wish to think, feel, and behave.* By letting go of your fear of experiencing life more fully, you can embrace and be more accepting of all your thoughts, beliefs, and emotions. This will allow you the joy of realizing your life's goals and the exhilaration of the unimpeded free flow of life-force energy. Remember, only through fully experiencing *both pain and joy* can you truly use your unique gifts and talents to thrive and fulfill your life purpose. And *if you can't feel it, you can't heal it.* This holds true for arthritis, sinusitis, heart problems, or any other chronic dis-ease. Your underlying emotional pain will be mirrored back to you with the ill health of your body and/or your mind. But so, too, will vitality and happiness reflect a condition of radiant health.

Chapter 6

HEALING YOUR SPIRIT

"What profit does a man receive if he gains the whole world only to lose his soul?"
MATTHEW 16:26

COMPONENTS OF OPTIMAL SPIRITUAL HEALTH

Experience of unconditional love/absence of fear

- Soul awareness and a personal relationship with God or Spirit
- Trusting your intuition and a willingness to change
- Gratitude
- Creating a sacred space on a regular basis through prayer, meditation, walking in nature, observing a Sabbath day, or other rituals
- Sense of purpose
- Being present in every moment.

The ultimate outcome of healing ourselves holistically is the recognition that we are truly spiritual beings, and the heightened awareness of the transcendent power known as God or Spirit. By making the commitment to become spiritually healthy, we open ourselves to the underlying life-force energy to which all religions refer and known in holistic medicine as *unconditional love*. Learning to love yourself in body, mind, and spirit is also the simplest and most direct way to learn to love God. To heal yourself spiritually means developing a relationship with Spirit in your own life and attuning yourself to Its guidance in all aspects of your daily existence. By doing so, you will begin to experience a profound reduction in your feelings of fear, and a greater capacity for loving yourself and others unconditionally. You will also become better able to identify your special talents and gifts and use them to fulfill your life's purpose *while fully experiencing the power of the present moment.*

In the deepest sense, all *dis-ease* can be seen as a disconnection between ourselves and Spirit, and a deprivation of love. From that perspective, spiritual health encompasses not only a conscious awareness of the Divine but also an intimate connection to ourselves, our families, our friends, and our communities. Just as mental health encompasses emotional health, spiritual health embraces social health. You cannot have one without the other. This truth is illustrated in the lives of the world's great spiritual teachers, including Moses, Jesus, Mohammed, Krishna, and Buddha, all of whom remained closely connected to their communities throughout the course of their ministries. Despite the apparent differences in their instructions to us, at their core, their messages are actually the same: *Place God first in all that you do, and love your neighbor as you love yourself.* As you reclaim your spiritual health, you fulfill their intention.

ACCESSING SPIRIT

"Every advance in knowledge brings us face to face with the mystery of our own being." Max Planck, father of quantum physics

You may believe that you are incapable of experiencing Spirit in your life, but that is not the case. *Spirit is present in any moment when we feel profoundly alive.* During these special moments, our predominant emotions are exhilaration and joy. The late Jesuit priest and scientist Pierre Teilhard de Chardin described *joy* as "the most infallible sign of the presence of God." Usually these fleeting moments surprise us: Our perception of reality is suddenly free of our normal judgments and concerns. Time seems to slow as we lose ourselves in *pure awareness.* Examples of these moments include experiencing the birth of your child, time spent with your beloved, being present at the death of someone you love, witnessing a sunset, entering "the zone" while playing sports, and being in the presence of inspirational works of art. Such peak experiences can also occur unexpectedly and spontaneously during the course of your normal routine, sparked by something as innocuous as hearing your favorite song on the radio. For most of us, these moments may seem to be accidental occurrences.

The purpose of this chapter is to help make your encounters with Spirit a more frequent and conscious part of your life. As you learn to master the techniques that follow, recognize that Spirit operates in much the same fashion as do subatomic particles: Both can be identified without being directly observed. Most often, and especially at the beginning of your spiritual journey, Spirit will be identified by the traces It leaves behind as It flows through you. With time and attention, each of us can deepen our perception of Spirit in our lives. Among the ways of doing so are *prayer, meditation, gratitude, spiritual practices, reconnecting with nature,* and *working with spiritual counselors.*

ARE WE SPIRITUAL BEINGS?
THE NEAR-DEATH EXPERIENCE

Most of us spend our lives deluded by the belief that our traits, habits, and actions are the sum total of who we are. In actuality these characteristic behaviors make up only our conscious personalities, or the sense of self that psychology refers to as the ego. Our ego is the source of our thoughts, judgments, and comparisons, which usually are based on past experience or future concerns. Largely fear-based, the ego diverts our attention from appreciating the reality that exists in the present moment. We live most of our waking hours in this ego state; yet, our true self, the soul (the individualized expression of Spirit), extends well beyond the limits of comprehension of the human intellect.

Letting go of the ego entails a surrender of mind and body that most of us equate with death. The thought of our death can be overpoweringly frightful. However, it is also one of the surest methods for reconnecting with our true spiritual natures. Every experience we have of transcendence and Spirit is also one in which we feel exhilarated and access a dimension of being beyond body and mind. If death is the freeing of our deeper self, or soul, from the physical plane, isn't it possible that it, too, can be an exhilarating experience? Certainly that is the report given by the vast majority of people who have had "near-death experiences." These episodes, also known as NDEs, involve people who were considered clinically dead in emergency or operating rooms, or at the scenes of accidents, and were subsequently resuscitated. In almost every case, these people report experiencing profound feelings of peace and unconditional love, as well as a reluctance to leave the spiritual dimension to return to their bodies.

The consistency of the reports of NDEs confirms the observation of many physicians and researchers who have scientifically studied the phenomena of death and dying that the soul remains intact beyond the death of the body. One of the leaders in this field is Elisabeth Kübler-Ross, M.D., who has pioneered this investigation for most of her professional career. After nearly thirty years of scientific research, she has concluded that "death does not exist . . . all that dies is a physical shell housing an immortal spirit." She also describes the time that we spend on earth as but a brief part of our total existence, and teaches that *to live well while we are here means to learn to love*—which is an active recognition, engagement, and appreciation of Spirit in ourselves and others. In one of her studies of over two hundred people who had experienced a near-death experience, almost all reported that they went before God and were asked the question, "How have you expanded your ability to give and receive love while you were down there?"

Whether or not you choose to believe the data being gathered in the fields of thanatology and NDE, there is mounting evidence strongly suggesting the existence of Spirit beyond the realms of mind and body. Choosing to believe this theory can heighten your creativity, enhance your healing capacity, free you to realize your life's purpose, diminish the level of fear in your life, and release the self-imposed limitations of past traumas. By becoming more aware of your soul—that part of yourself that does not die—you will be better able to take risks and pursue the dreams of your life.

PRAYER

The most common form of spiritual exercise engaged in by most Americans is prayer. Nearly 90 percent of us pray, and 70 percent of us believe that prayer can lead to physical, emotional, or spiritual healing. Most people who pray have a greater sense of well-being than those who don't, and, when polled, the majority of people who pray say that through prayer they experience a sense of peace, receive answers to life issues, and have even felt divinely inspired or "led by God" to perform some specific action. Interestingly, people who experience a "sense of the Divine" during prayer also score the highest on ratings of general well-being and satisfaction with their lives.

In recent years, a great deal of scientific study has focused on the beneficial effects of prayer. Among the studies is one by the National Institute of Mental Health in 1994, which examined nearly three thousand North Carolinians and found that those who attended church weekly had 29 percent less risk of alcoholism than those who attended less frequently. In the same study, the risk of alcoholism decreased by 42 percent among those who prayed and read the Bible regularly. Another NIMH study conducted in the same year found that frequent churchgoers also had lower rates of depression and other mental problems.

An examination of 212 medical studies examining the relationship between religious beliefs and health by Dale A. Matthews, M.D., associate professor of medicine at Georgetown University, found that 75 percent of the studies showed health benefits for those patients with "religious commitments." Among patients with hypertension, regular prayer reduced blood pressure in 50 percent of all cases.

Among the pioneers in the study of the physiological effects of prayer and meditation is Herbert Benson, M.D., a Harvard cardiologist. In 1968, Benson began studying people who regularly practiced transcendental meditation (TM). The subjects meditated by focusing on a mantra, such as *Om,* that had no apparent meaning to its user. Benson discovered that repetition of the mantra resulted in a lower metabolic rate, slower heart rate, lower blood pressure, and slower breathing. He dubbed this physiological effect the *relaxation response.* Benson then turned his attention to Christians and Jews who prayed instead of meditating, instructing them to repeat religious phrases such as the first line of the Lord's Prayer, "Hail Mary, full of grace," "The Lord is my shepherd," or "Shalom." He found that the phrases all produced the same relaxation response that is triggered by meditation, and that the degree of physiological benefit is determined by the degree of faith on the part of the person praying.

Since 1988, Benson and psychologist Jared Klass have been conducting a series of programs at the Mind/Body Medical Institute at New England Deaconess Hospital, inviting priests, rabbis, and ministers to investigate the spiritual and health implications of prayer. In their studies, a psychological scale developed by Benson and Klass for measuring spirituality is employed. People scoring high in spirituality—defined by Benson as a feeling that "there is more than just you" and as not necessarily religious—score higher in psychological health. They also:

- were less likely to get sick, and were better able to cope if they did
- had fewer stress-related symptoms
- gained the most from meditation training
- showed the greatest rise on a life-purpose index
- Exhibited the sharpest drop in pain.

To begin the practice of prayer, start with any prayer you are comfortable with or recall from your religious training as a child. You can also use a favorite psalm or passage from the Bible or prayer book you find especially meaningful. In addition you can engage in personal prayer, talking to God as if you were speaking to your best friend. State your need or concern and ask for God's help. (It is more effective to pray for the peace that would result from having what you desire, than pray for the specific things themselves.) Whichever form of prayer you choose, try to establish a regular routine and repeat your prayer morning and night.

MEDITATION

In the West, meditation has primarily been studied for its mental, emotional, and physiological benefits, while in the East it has primarily been used for thousands of years to still the mind in order to heighten awareness and contact soul and Spirit. During meditation, practitioners enter into a neutral emotional state, becoming a witness to their passing thoughts and feelings as they move into a state of heightened attention that can ultimately result in pure awareness.

As with prayer, there are many ways to meditate. Meditation can be performed while sitting or in a supine position, or while on the move—walking, jogging, and even during sports. What all forms of meditation have in common is a focusing on the breath and an emptying of the mind of thought. With regular practice, meditators typically report increased feelings of calm and peace, improved mental functioning and enhanced powers of concentration, and a deeper connection to Spirit, which is often perceived as a quiet, inner voice guiding them in their actions. Other reported benefits include increased equanimity toward, and detachment from, life events; increased energy and joy; feelings of bliss and ecstasy; and increased dream recall.

It is best to learn meditation under the guidance of a qualified instructor, but a variety of books and audiotapes are also available on the subject. The simplest method of meditation is to sit in a quiet place, resting comfortably in a chair, with your spine erect and your feet flat on the floor. Close your eyes and begin focusing on your breathing, keeping your awareness on each inhalation and exhalation. To improve your concentration, you may wish to silently repeat the word *in* as you inhale, and *out* as you exhale. Or you can repeat a word or mantra, such as *love, peace, God, Om,* or *Hu* (both latter terms are names for the Divine). Allow your thoughts to come and go without lingering on them, as if your awareness were a running stream and your thoughts were simply leaves floating by. At first you may feel deluged with thoughts. Each time you find yourself distracted, simply bring your attention back to your breathing. Eventually you may notice longer periods of silence between each thought. It may take months to quiet your mind to this extent, but with consistent practice your meditation *will* become deeper and easier. Try to sit for at least ten minutes once or twice a day, gradually working up to two half-hour sessions per day. It's important to keep your practice regular and consistent, but don't force things. If you find yourself too distracted or pressed for time, end your session until next time instead of sitting restlessly.

Walking meditation is another form of meditation that in recent years has been popularized by the Buddhist monk Thich Nhat Hanh. This means of meditation is often suited for active people who find it difficult to sit still. The goal is to focus your attention in the present by focusing on each step you take in tandem with your breathing. To enhance your experience, you can mentally repeat *With each step I take I am fully present to my surroundings.* Over time, as you practice this form of meditation, don't be surprised if you find it becomes more difficult to hurry. The more you focus on the present, the less consequence time has as you discover how profound even a simple act such as walking can be.

GRATITUDE

Most religious traditions prescribe specific prayers or grace before meals as a way of thanking God for our food and sustenance. As with other spiritual practices, there is something to be gained from these rituals or they wouldn't have survived for thousands of years. A sense of gratitude for all the other areas of our lives can elicit similar life-enhancing benefits.

Gratitude has been called the "Great Attitude." Although most of us tend to take our lives for granted, they are in fact a gift, and every day that we are alive each of us receives many blessings. Even times of pain and adversity, such as suffering with arthritis, can be seen as opportunities for growth for which we can be grateful. By committing ourselves to becoming more aware of our blessings, we strengthen our connection with Spirit and are able to better recognize the wisdom and intelligence that underlies all of creation.

Once we allow ourselves to appreciate the lessons presented during times of struggle or life crises, the brunt of the pain subsides and a state of inner peace follows. This is especially true of most chronic diseases, which can be seen as external reflections of inner (emotional and/or spiritual) pain. Typically, when people choose to consciously focus on the positives in their lives and express gratitude for them, more positive things start to happen. For instance, while you're learning to live with your arthritis, suppose you spent time each day focusing on the blessings and the many pleasures your body has provided you with in the past along with the multitude of basic functions for which it still serves you well. These include the ability to breathe fully, to make love, and to enjoy eating, drinking, digesting, and eliminating. You may not have the ability or energy to exercise as you once did, but you can still relish the peacefulness of a quiet walk in nature. You've still retained the capacity to choose your beliefs and attitudes, as well as to experience, express, and accept all of your feelings. In addition, this physical disability can serve as a powerful catalyst for becoming better acquainted with your soul and Spirit. You may have never recognized the spiritual being that you truly are, or your purpose for being here, had you not been blessed with arthritis. This may sound unreasonable or even irrational to you, but it was certainly helpful to me in curing my chronic sinusitis. For many years I suffered and felt as if I were cursed. I angrily asked of God, "Why me? What have I done to deserve this misery?" Yet, now I can clearly see how this physical pain has so enriched my life. It's taught me how to give and receive love—to nurture my body, home and work environments, mind, emotional body, intimate relationships, and my soul. This is the essence of the work I came here to do, and it has become my full-time job. I call it training to thrive, and at 53, I'm healthier and more fit physically, mentally, and spiritually than I've ever been. Who knows what my life would have been like had I not been blessed with sinusitis, or yours without arthritis.

Gratitude can produce powerful feelings of joy and self-acceptance, and is an attitude that anyone can choose to have, just as you can choose to see the glass half full or half empty. By focusing on what you do have instead of what you lack, you feel a sense of abundance that makes your problems seem much less acute, and you are better able to let go of negative thoughts and attitudes. This usually isn't easy to do, especially if you are feeling a great deal of fear or anger. But if you make the effort to release these painful emotions and *choose the attitude of gratitude,* even for a moment, wonderful things can happen.

Like any habit, that of recognizing and acknowledging the gifts in your life requires practice. One simple way to begin feeling grateful is the following visualization taught by Rabbi Mordecai Twerski, the spiritual leader of Denver's Hasidic community. As soon as you wake up each morning, before you get out of bed, close your eyes and picture a person, scene, or situation that made you happy to be alive and for which you are still grateful. You never would have had that experience if you weren't alive, and by allowing yourself to reexperience it, you open yourself up to the awareness that something equally wonderful can happen today. Create the habit of practicing this visualization each morning upon awakening and you will soon instill in yourself a new attitude of anticipation and appreciation for the day ahead.

Another way to cultivate feelings of gratitude is by making a *gratitude list.* This exercise is best performed before going to bed, as a way to detach yourself from any concerns or problems you may have in order to appreciate the gifts and lessons that came your way during the day. Some people prefer to write out their list; others simply close their eyes and mentally review their day, making themselves aware of all the things that happened for which they feel grateful. Either way works well. Complete the exercise by praying silently, giving thanks for all that you experienced and learned that day.

By making gratitude a regular part of your daily experience, you set the stage for living more deeply connected to Spirit. In the process, your life will be transformed into an increasingly joyous adventure.

INTUITION

As you progress in your healing journey, eventually you will find yourself being guided by your intuition, which is often experienced as an "inner nudge" or a "still, quiet voice" speaking from within. If you are not already aware of your intuitive messages, most likely it is because your intuition is having a tough time competing for your attention. Most of the inner messages you hear come from your ego and tend to be loud, self-centered, and fear-based. Intuitive messages, by contrast, come from the heart and are usually more subtle, compassionate, energizing, and enlivening.

In order to develop your sense of intuition, you will need to slow down, eliminate distractions, and do a lot less talking. The methods provided in this chapter can help you to do so. Slow, relaxing walks are another helpful way to make contact with this inner guidance. The next step is learning to recognize when your intuition is truly speaking to you, and when it is not. Learning to discern the difference requires practice. One useful method for determining if the "voice" you hear is indeed your intuition is to notice how it feels. Often intuitive messages occur accompanied by feelings of excitement or an unequivocal sense that acting upon them is "the right thing to do." People who haven't learned to trust their intuition often experience doubts or fears immediately following such feelings. "How can I be sure this is true?" "What if I'm wrong?" These and similar questions can quickly quash your inner guidance if you haven't learned to trust it.

To help you know if the messages you receive are in your best interest, experiment with the following exercise. Out loud, tell yourself something that you know to be true. As you do so, notice how you feel. Now state aloud something you know to be false. Again notice how you feel. Usually people practicing this exercise experience feelings of discomfort, confusion, even pain, in their bodies when they make the false statement, whereas they feel in alignment with the statement that is true. (Often the sensations occur in the area of the solar plexus, with false statements provoking queasy feelings or tension.)

Allowing yourself to be guided by your intuition is ultimately an act of faith. At first, learning to trust and act on the intuitive messages you receive will involve risk. The more trust you bring to your practice, however, the easier it will be to take action. Realize, too, that sometimes the results of following your intuition may be painful. Such times are not necessarily mistakes. They can be seen as lessons teaching you how to listen more effectively. Or they may be necessary to facilitate your growth and help you to better understand the higher purpose toward which Spirit is guiding you.

SPIRITUAL COUNSELORS

Due to the many uncertainties that can be part of the spiritual journey, you may consider working with a spiritual counselor, especially if you haven't been in the habit of listening to your intuition or need help in "tuning in" to Spirit. Just as you would visit a doctor to heal your physical body, or a psychotherapist to heal mental and emotional issues, spiritual counselors can help connect you to your spiritual core. The most common resources for spiritual counseling are priests, rabbis, ministers, and other clergy. Spiritual psychotherapists, medical intuitives, clairvoyants, and spiritual healers or shamans can also be of great assistance.

What these healers have in common is an ability to see beyond the boundaries of the five senses. Their services may include helping you to identify your life purpose, pointing out opportunities for your spiritual growth, or scanning your body's bioenergy field to diagnose the underlying cause of a particular health condition. Their primary value, however, lies in the assistance they can provide in helping you appreciate the meaning and lessons of your daily life, especially those that are most painful.

Because of the lack of certification in these areas, to find a spiritual counselor, you may need to rely upon references from people you trust, experience some trial and error, and call upon your own intuition. Keep an open mind and see how you respond to the information provided. Some of these counselors are truly gifted and can provide you with information that can be a catalyst for transforming your life.

SPIRITUAL PRACTICES

Most of us have some sort of spiritual orientation, even if it is no more than what we received in childhood. Yet, we often fail to realize how much some of these practices can contribute to our health. The ritual observance of *Sabbath,* for instance, can be an enormously healing experience, as it restores the sacred rhythm between work and rest. We're so busy *doing* in our society that we've forgotten how to just *be* and appreciate the delight of simply being alive. The Sabbath day is also a particularly good time to practice gratitude as you contemplate the blessings you share with those you love. Studies also reveal that those who regularly observe a weekly holy day tend to score higher in areas of optimism, stress management, and general well-being.

Fasting is another spiritual practice that is also healing. Not only can fasting have a cleansing effect upon the body, eliminating toxins while giving the organs of digestion and assimilation a rest, it can also elicit a heightened feeling of spirituality and result in the healing of old emotional wounds. In his book *Live Better Longer,* Joseph Dispenza, director of the Parcells Center in

Santa Fe, New Mexico, points out that fasting can purge the emotional body of old, toxic feelings, facilitate the release of psychological patterns that no longer work for you, and "open your mind and heart to new emotional, psychological, and spiritual sustenance." (The Parcells Center is based on the work of Dr. Hazel Parcells, a scientist and naturopathic physician who, at 41, cured herself of terminal tuberculosis using fasts and other natural methods. She then went on to live a life of vibrant, robust health until she died peacefully in her sleep at age 106.)

If you are new to fasting, try a twenty-four-hour fast, selecting a day when work and other responsibilities are limited and you won't be too active. Plan for some quiet time alone and, during the final two hours of the fast, drink six to eight glass of water to help cleanse your body of toxins.

Gabriel Cousens, M.D., at his Tree of Life Rejuvenation Center in Patagonia, Arizona, has had great success in treating a variety of diseases, including arthritis, diabetes, alcoholism, and asthma, with fasting and meditation.

The potential that spiritual practices have to heal is illustrated in the case of one of my friend and colleague Dr. Bob Anderson's patients, a 64-year-old woman named Lois, who underwent the surgical removal of a very large, aggressive ovarian cancer. The procedure left her with a colostomy, and part of the original tumor was not removable, leaving hundreds of small metastases throughout her abdominal cavity. On Dr. Anderson's insistence, Lois agreed to consult with an oncologist, only to promptly reject his recommendation of chemotherapy despite the fact that remnants of her tumor remained in her pelvis and abdomen. She was convinced that her condition would be cured by her own body with God's help, and returned to Dr. Anderson to aid her in getting well. Although she undertook many initiatives, central to her program was her faith in the power of prayer and God. Each day she meditated for up to an hour and prayed numerous times.

Four months later Lois was finally able to persuade her surgeon to remove the colostomy to restore her internal bowel function. During the course of a long and tedious surgery, hundreds of small, metastasized tumors appeared as before. Seven of them were biopsied. Three days later the pathology report showed that their cancerous characteristics were gone. Lois fully recovered and resumed an active life focused around the activities she enjoyed and her continued prayers to God. Two years later an operation to repair an abdominal hernia revealed that her abdomen and pelvis were completely normal, with no residual cancer anywhere. Although he has no way of proving it, Dr. Anderson remains convinced that Lois's daily prayers and meditations were somehow central to her recovery.

Finding Spirit in Nature

Nowhere is the creative power of Spirit more visible than in nature. It is here that we most directly experience life's four elemental forms of energy: earth, water, fire, and air. Earth is matter in its deepest form; water represents the receptive yielding principle; fire is the transformational energy that causes matter to change form; and air is the resultant blend of these other three elements into a subtler vibration of life-force energy. In our bodies, earth is cellular matter, water is blood and circulation, fire is metabolism and energy production, and air is oxygen, the nutrient most essential for our sustenance. By regularly exposing yourself to nature's four elements—ideally on a daily basis—you will expand your awareness of how each of them is uniquely embodied within you and more fully appreciate the healing power of nature. What follows are ways for you to do so.

Earth. Spend as much time as possible outdoors in close contact with the earth. Walking is a wonderful way to do this, as are outdoor sports, bike rides in a park, and gardening. When you can, also visit the beach, woods, and mountains, and take time to notice the beauty surrounding you. The more time you spend immersed nature, the more aware you will become of life's natural rhythms and the ways the earth retains and radiates energy.

As a society, we need to recognize that cities and other industrialized areas are in fact unnatural and can keep us from living a life of balance. Making the effort to spend time in nature can go a long way to restoring that balance while deepening your connection with Spirit at the same time.

Water. One of the most visible forms of Spirit in nature is the flow of water as it follows the contours of the earth. Water is a receptive form of energy and is affected by the forces acting upon it. Rivers flow, for example, due to the gravitational pull caused by the gradient of the landscape. The action of water tumbling over rocks also releases a more subtle energy in the form of negative ions, which can contribute to feelings of well-being. Swimming in the ocean, lakes, or rivers provides invaluable exposure to this special form of energy. Soaking in a mineral hot spring can also provide therapeutic benefits for a variety of ailments, and can be one of life's great pleasures.

A healthy routine that anyone can adopt is bathing in warm water at least once a day. For added benefit, practice conscious breathing while you enjoy a soak in the tub. This is a very effective way to connect with your body's bioenergy field, and can help heal mental and emotional upset.

Fire. Throughout the Bible and other sacred scriptures, the dominant symbols of the divine essence in human beings is fire and light, such as the tale of Moses speaking to God in the burning bush, or the transfiguration of Jesus on the mountaintop before his closest apostles. Candlelight is also common as a tool for spiritual focus in most religions. Anyone who has experienced the pleasures of an open campfire can attest to the healing properties of fire. According to Leonard Orr, the founder of Rebirthing, spending time before an open fire, including a fireplace, cleanses the bioenergy field of negative energies and can be a powerful aid in curing physical disease. Orr recommends spending a few hours each day before fire for people who want to experience such benefits.

Fire is also an important component of the vision quests employed by Native Americans as a means of connecting to Spirit and discerning their life purpose. The ultimate source of fire energy is the sun, which provides healing and creative energy that directly or indirectly gives life to all living organisms. Regular exposure to sunlight has been linked to a variety of mental and emotional benefits, while depression, anxiety, and other mental *dis-ease* can occur when we are deprived of the sun's healing rays (e.g. Seasonal Affective Disorder, or SAD). Time spent daily in the sun is a very healthy practice as long as appropriate precautions are taken, including sunscreen, hats, and long sleeves and pants when needed.

Air. Of the four elements, air is perhaps the closest expression of Spirit, so much so that the ancient Greeks equated Spirit (pneuma) with the wind. The most potent method of imbuing yourself with the life-force energy of air is through meditation and other forms of conscious breathing. A daily practice of these methods can significantly energize you, open you up to new levels of creativity and productivity, and make you more aware of Spirit's guidance and power flowing through you.

SOCIAL HEALTH

"No man is an island." John Donne

Components of Optimal Social Health

Intimacy with a spouse, partner, relative, or close friend

- Effective communication
- Forgiveness
- Touch and/or physical intimacy on a daily basis
- Sense of belonging to a support group or community
- Selflessness and altruism.

Our relationships with others is the crucible that most determines how spiritually healthy we are. Optimal *social health* consists of a strong positive connection to others in community and family, and intimacy with one or more people. It is often much easier to feel our connection with Spirit during moments of solitude than it is to express that connection through our interactions with others. At the same time, our relationships offer us the greatest opportunities for spiritual growth and for learning how to receive and impart unconditional love. *True spiritual health is a balance between the autonomy of the self and intimacy with others.*

The importance of social relationships, love, and intimacy with respect to health is documented in a growing number of studies demonstrating the benefits of the diversity and depth of connection to community, family, and spouse. Lack of healthy social relationships is a common denominator among patients with heart disease, particularly when accompanied by feelings of hostility and a sense of isolation. Conversely, the longevity of terminal cancer patients with long-term survival rates has been attributed to a relatively high degree of social involvement. One of the most convincing studies highlighting the importance of community showed that Hispanics, despite poverty, lack of health insurance, and poor access to medical care, are surprisingly less likely than whites to die of major chronic diseases, including all forms of cancer, heart disease, and respiratory ailments. Further, with the exception of diabetes, liver disease, and homicide, their overall health outlook is significantly better than for whites. Some health experts, including former Surgeon General Antonia Coello Novello, the first Latina to serve in that post, postulate that the reason for this stems from Hispanic culture, which promotes strong family values and frowns on health risks such as drinking and smoking. Based on a growing number of relationship studies, researchers have concluded that *social isolation is statistically just as dangerous as smoking, high blood pressure, high cholesterol, obesity, or lack of exercise.*

The primary opportunities available to each of us for improving our social health include forgiveness, friendships, selfless acts and altruism, support groups, and especially marriage, committed relationships, and parenting.

Forgiveness

"To err is human; to forgive, divine."   ALEXANDER POPE

Intimate relationships and unconditional love cannot exist without forgiveness. How often do you blame yourself for your past actions and mistakes? How often do you blame others for your own problems, stress, or slights (both real and imagined) against you? Forgiveness cancels the demands that you or others *should* have done things differently. Hanging on to these demands changes nothing but keeps us under stress. Refusing to forgive yourself or others keeps you locked into limiting patterns from your past, unable to mobilize the creative power in your life here and now.

The next time you find yourself blaming others, physically point your index finger at them or their images and take a look at where the other three fingers of your hand are pointed. Right back at you! Forgiveness, therefore, begins with accepting responsibility for the role you play in shaping your life's experiences. Only after you begin to forgive yourself can you truly forgive others.

A key first step in your journey of forgiveness is the recognition that you are always doing the best you can at any given moment, in accordance with your awareness at the time. This is true of everyone else as well. All of us make mistakes, and all of us ideally learn from them. You may even choose to believe that there are no mistakes, only lessons. In that moment your action or behavior was based upon past experience, environment, and heredity. You can, however, consciously choose to be different in the future. To continue to blame yourself or someone else for something that occurred in the past is energy depleting and keeps you from moving forward with your life.

Forgiving yourself may be your greatest challenge. No doubt there are a number of things in your past that you regret or for which you feel shame. But wouldn't it be healthier to look at what you can learn from your mistake or painful lesson so that it's not repeated; forgive yourself unconditionally for not knowing more or not performing well enough; and be grateful for this opportunity to learn to do better or change your behavior? A tennis player who misses a shot he thinks he should have made will lose his confidence and ultimately his match if he doesn't quickly recognize what he did wrong, forgive himself, and move on to play the next point. Similarly we lose the ability to focus and do as well as we know we are capable of doing in the present if we do not forgive ourselves and let go of the past.

The more you are able to do this for yourself, the better you will be able to forgive others. *Remember, you are forgiving the actor, not the action.* You are not condoning cruelty, insensitivity, or incompetence; you are forgiving the offending person. By doing so, you are freeing yourself to move out of the past into the healing present. Anger is the problem; forgiveness is the solution.

Bear in mind, however, that the people you decide to forgive may not choose to accept your forgiveness. Although their refusal to do so can be hurtful, their choice should be respected. What matters is that you are taking the step to heal the relationship. The act of forgiveness takes place within your own psyche, and the person you are forgiving may therefore be totally unaware of your action. Or you may be forgiving someone who is deceased. Be realistic and don't set your sights too high: Begin with someone who has been critical of you or guilty of another relatively minor offense. Forgiving others does not necessarily mean that your relationship with them will change, but forgiving them will enable you to feel a greater sense of wholeness. Your relationship with the people you forgive may remain the same on the surface, but it doesn't mean that healing hasn't taken place. You will know it when you feel it.

Friendship

A 1997 study from Carnegie Mellon University in Pittsburgh found that people with a greater diversity of relationships were less likely to get colds. Those with six or more social ties (family, friends, co-workers, neighbors, etc.) were four times *less* susceptible to colds than those with one to three types of relationships. Researchers found that it was not the number of people in the social network that was the important factor, but the diversity. To varying degrees, most of these types of relationships can be called *friendships.*

As children and teenagers, most of us had a number of friends with whom we enjoyed sharing the day's adventures. Our friends helped us meet such challenges as starting each new school year, participating in sports, going through puberty, dating, dealing with family problems, and getting through the existential concerns that all of us face throughout our journey into adulthood. Between kindergarten and college, sustaining friendships was made easier by the fact that our friends provided us with a sense of belonging, a feeling of "being in this together," and offered us a forum in which to mutually discuss the problems and issues we faced at the time. Because of such friendships, many people regard the times they spent in high school and college as the happiest days of their lives. Once past college, as they entered the workforce, got married, and juggled the responsibilities of their careers and families, a large segment of our society has lost track of their friends from the past and have not replaced them with new friends.

While most adults enjoy the company of neighbors, co-workers, and other acquaintances, by the time we reach our thirties, studies reveal that those of us who still have a best friend in whom we can confide are exceptionally rare. This is particularly true of men who, because of this lack of a confidant, experience feelings of isolation and absence of support, no matter how fulfilled they may otherwise be in their personal lives and careers.

If you find yourself in need of a good friend, realize that it's never too late to rekindle old friendships or to make new ones. All that is required is a willingness to take risks and make the effort. Having a close friend you can talk to from your heart can provide many additional blessings in your life and deepen your connection with Spirit.

Selfless Acts and Altruism

Remember a time when you stopped to spontaneously help someone, either a friend or a total stranger? Such selfless acts of giving go to the essence of Spirit, which is always with us, supporting our lives while asking for nothing in return. *Sharing* with others your time, help, and special gifts and talents in ways that benefit them provides you with perhaps the most powerful means of engaging and expressing Spirit and enhancing social health. The opportunities for sharing are abundant and may include donating clothes or money to worthy charities, volunteering time at a homeless shelter, soup kitchen, or after-school tutoring program, or simply setting aside our own tasks and concerns to address the needs of our spouses or children. (There is a great deal of truth is the adage "Charity begins at home.") Another form of sharing that is regaining popularity is *tithing*. Dating back to biblical times, tithing is the practice of donating a certain percentage (usually 5 to 10 percent) of one's yearly income to charity. Interestingly, many people who adopt the practice of tithing also find that their incomes actually begin to increase, although that should not be your motivation for doing so. However you choose to perform selfless acts, remember that the truest form of giving is one that does not call attention to the giver. As Jesus instructed in the Gospel of Matthew, "When you give to the needy, do not announce it with trumpets." The purpose of sharing is *to share,* not to acquire praise or honors. Sharing selflessly will deepen your awareness of how abundantly Spirit is giving to you.

The late Hans Selye, a pioneer in modern stress research, thought that by helping people you earn their gratitude and affection, and that the warmth that results protects against stress. Today, Selye's belief is borne out by mounting evidence that selfless acts not only feel good but are healthy. Epidemiologist James House and his colleagues at the University of Michigan's Survey Research Center studied more than 2,700 men in Tecumseh, Michigan, for almost fourteen years to see how social relationships affected mortality rates. Those who did regular volunteer work had death rates two-and-one-half times lower than those who didn't. The highest form of selfishness is selflessness. When we freely choose to help others, we seem to get as much, or more, than what we give.

The closer our contact with those we help, the greater the benefits seem to be. Most of us need to feel that we matter to someone, a need that volunteer work can fulfill. There is a growing number of people requiring help in our society, including the homeless, the elderly, the hungry, runaways, orphans, and the illiterate, and there are many ways to help them. Choose to do so in the way that most compels you, but recognize that altruism works best when it comes from the heart and is not calculated as a means to receive something in return.

Support Groups

As a society we are plagued by social ills, most notably divorce rates that top 50 percent, a general sentiment of feeling overworked, dual-career marriages, increasing single-parent families, and a generation of children more adrift and alone than any that has preceded them. At the same time a movement is afoot in America toward a greater sense of community in response to the silent epidemic of isolation and loneliness that affects so many of us. As a result there has been a significant increase in support groups for those sharing common values, experiences, and goals. Support groups for couples, divorced people, single parents, men, women, people with an illness in common (especially cancer), and people recovering from alcohol and drug addiction—and other addictions—are gathering all over the country. Many of them are affiliated with a church or synagogue, with the added purpose of enhancing spiritual growth. They meet regularly—weekly, every other week, or every month—and the participants by and large report that they benefit from the social connection they find there. If you would like to participate in such a group, most likely you can find them in your local Yellow Pages, or you can contact organizations such as your local United Way, Catholic Charities, AA group, etc. Many communities also have support groups devoted to specific diseases, and can also be found on the Internet.

Recent scientific research also verifies that support groups can play an important role in helping people with chronic disease. David Spiegel, M.D., conducted a study at Stanford University School of Medicine on women with metastatic breast cancer. All of the women received chemotherapy or radiation therapy. One half of them were in a support group that met weekly for one year. These women lived twice as long as those who were not in a support group, and three were still alive ten years later.

Committed Relationships and Marriage

Healthy committed relationships promote physical, emotional, and especially spiritual well-being through the experience of unconditional love. The model for all committed relationships is marriage, usually the most challenging as well as the most rewarding of all interpersonal relationships. It is potentially our most powerful spiritual practice. If humanity's fundamental moral principle is "Love thy neighbor as thyself," its practice begins not with the person living next door but with the neighbor with whom we share our bed.

Regardless of who your partner may be or how long you have been involved with him or her, the key to all committed relationships is *intimacy*. Think of intimacy as *into-me-see*. As you develop the skills for seeing into—and learning to appreciate—yourself, you have the opportunity to also "see into" your partner and allow your partner to see into you. Once a commitment is made, the relationship becomes greater than the sum of its parts, allowing both partners to flourish and realize their full potential as human beings. The transformation that can occur in marriage and other committed relationships is primarily a result of letting go of judgment. As you do so, you will realize that in giving more to the relationship you are ultimately giving to yourself. Studies have shown that you may otherwise be contributing to making yourself and your partner sick. Marital conflict lowers immune function, especially in women, according to researchers at Ohio State University.

Hallmarks of a healthy committed relationship include having a shared vision, attentive listening to each other, the freedom to make requests so that both partners can better ensure that their needs are met, and regular intervals of fun and recreation together. If you are interested in making a deeper commitment to your relationship, you might also consider working with a good marriage counselor or other relationship teacher.

Shared Vision. A vision that you share with your partner is a way of defining your mutual goals and focusing your energy on their attainment. Lack of a vision can cause your relationship to lose direction or become stagnant. One simple but effective way to create a shared vision with your spouse or partner is to take time to individually list your relationship goals (keep them positive, short, descriptive, specific), prioritizing them in numerical order. Then begin combining lists, starting with the goals having the highest value and alternating between the two lists to form a composite vision you and your partner are both comfortable with. The resulting "mutual relationship vision" can help keep you and your partner working together toward your common goals while reducing conflict and enhancing your relationship.

Attentive listening. Most of us are poor listeners: We *hear* what is being said, but we don't always *listen* to it. This is because hearing can be unconscious, while listening requires conscious effort. Since communication is the foundation of any relationship, and listening is a critical aspect of effective communication, it is important to get in the habit of consciously paying attention to what your partner tells you *without responding immediately.* The practice of listening can greatly enhance both intimacy and autonomy. This type of listening can be practiced as a "listening exercise." Schedule an uninterrupted forty-minute block of time in which both you and your partner speak for twenty minutes while the other person listens *without responding.* Talk only about yourself and how you're feeling, without blaming or talking about your relationship issues. There is no discussion following the exercise.

Attentive listening makes it possible for both partners to be able to talk freely and express thoughts and feelings without worrying about judgment or criticism. Focusing on what your partner is saying requires you to empty your mind of your own thoughts and concerns as you listen, thereby minimizing negative reactions. This exercise allows for a balance between intimacy and autonomy, a critical component of healthy relationships. Cultivating the habit of attentive listening will help you and your partner create a safe environment for expressing your feelings, allowing you to be more vulnerable and open with each other, which is extremely valuable for building trust, understanding, and deeper, even exhilarating, feelings of intimacy.

Requests. By committing to another person, you enter into a relationship in which you have promised to give and receive love. But since each of us is different, what feels like love to one person may not even be noticed by another. Most of us attempt to love our partners in ways that feel like love to *us,* and are surprised when they do not react as we would. A good method for eliminating this problem is simply to tell the other what feels good to you and what you want.

It can be quite a revelation when someone you thought you knew well tells you what they really *need* from you. We often expect our partners to be able to read our minds, but we really can't know what each other wants unless we are told. Refrain from general statements such as "Love me" or "Be nice to me." Making specific requests like "I would like you to buy me flowers once a week" or "I would like you to cook dinner once a week" will significantly improve the likelihood that you will get what you need. When you do, be sure to thank your partner for complying with your request. This is extremely important, since your request is usually not an easy or natural thing for your partner to do. Otherwise you probably wouldn't have had to ask for it in the first place.

Having fun together. Life's daily pressures and responsibilities make it difficult to remember to have fun. For many couples, the glue that reinforces their relationship is the memory of the enjoyment they shared during their courtship and early years together. Setting aside time that you and your partner can spend in recreation together is an important way to *re-create* the joy and spontaneity that first brought you together. To rekindle some of that excitement and minimize the risk of boring routines, it helps to schedule fun activities together on a regular basis. Plan at least half a day each week to spend together away from home, taking turns each time to choose your activity. Getting out of the house, alone together, can help you focus attention on each other. Although this is more difficult to do if you have young children, it is still possible to plan an exciting evening at home after they go to bed. Choose something neither of you has tried before to add another dimension of adventure to your play, and, if you can manage it, plan several weekends per year out of town. This can be especially rewarding if a real vacation isn't feasible. Having fun regularly with the person you love is refreshing and invigorating, and can help ensure that your relationship remains healthy and fulfilling.

Sex

Of all the major world religions, the Judeo-Christian tradition is the only one that does not commonly recognize the potential that sexual intercourse has as a pathway to Spirit. Other religions, including Hinduism, Buddhism, Islam, and Taoism, as well as the spiritual traditions of Africa and the Amerindians, freely acknowledge that sex, properly entered into, can be a powerful spiritual experience capable of transforming consciousness and enhancing physical and emotional health.

In the West, perhaps the most well-known of these teachings on sex is *tantra*. This is an ancient system of sexual and sensual techniques for consciously controlling the mind, increasing life-force energy, and tapping into Spirit. Tantra's erotic practices include specific positions, breath, and visualization to heighten sexual energy and move it upward along the spine in order to create rapturous waves of blissful energy that can ultimately lead to enlightenment. Many mystic writings, such as the verse of the Sufi poet-saint Rumi, also refer to the Divine using the language of sex and romantic love, often equating God with the Beloved while yearning to experience union with the Absolute.

To experience sex from this exalted perspective requires expanding your focus beyond physical gratification and genital orgasm, into an experience of yourself and your spouse or lover as expressions of Spirit-in-the-flesh. Adopting this attitude leaves you extremely vulnerable and simultaneously in touch with your own divine power. Lovemaking in this state is free of the machinations of ego and proceeds slowly, gently, and consciously, ensuring that the needs of both partners are always met before moving on to the next cycle of pleasure and awareness. Couples who master this approach are able to remain in a state of heightened excitation for several hours, prolong and intensify orgasm, and experience total body orgasms. Among the experiences they report are a continuous flow of energy throughout their bodies, a joined climax of body and soul, the sensation of being united with the cosmos, and, afterward, being refreshed and revitalized. The primary goal of "spiritual sex" isn't prolonged orgasm, however, but an experience of being more deeply connected with the person you love and, through that connectedness, having an awareness of your integral role within the whole of creation. Not everyone will feel the need to master, or even explore, a tantric approach to sex; yet, all of us can benefit from more conscious lovemaking. Of all the spiritual practices, it is certainly the most pleasurable. (To learn more about the tantric approach to sex, see *The Art of Sexual Ecstasy* by Margo Anand.)

Parenting

Parenting is easily one of life's most enriching experiences and, at the same time, one of our most challenging jobs. Through their children, parents have the opportunity to reconnect with play, to feel more in touch with their own "inner child," to experience selflessness, and to learn how to love unconditionally. Those of us who are parents are also provided with a wonderful forum for practicing forgiveness, trust, acceptance of ourselves and others, self-awareness, and, most of all, patience (as any parent of a teenager well knows). Perhaps the greatest human expression of love is that of parents for their children.

Unfortunately, in our society parenting isn't always consciously approached. If you are already a parent, however, it is not too late to meet your parental obligations more consciously than you may currently be doing. One useful guideline is to regularly ask yourself: *Will this [action, response, activity, demand] of mine help my child's self-esteem?* The same principle holds true in parenting as it does in marriage: *To love another is to help that person better love him- or herself.* This commitment will not only affect your child's happiness in the present but will significantly impact his or her future health. In the landmark Harvard Mastery of Stress Study, college students rated their parents on their level of parental caring. Thirty-five years later, 87 percent of those who rated both parents low on parental love suffered from a chronic illness, whereas only 25 percent of those who rated both parents high in caring had a disease.

In the field of family therapy, the family is usually seen as a "system." This view holds that if a family member's behavior is harmful to himself or others, the problem and the solution lie not only within the individual but within the entire family system. This perspective encourages parents to examine their roles and the responsibility they share with their child for his or her problem. Often, a child's crisis serves as a mirror reflecting an imbalance in his or her individual system as well as in the family system as a whole. One of the significant advantages of family therapy is that change often occurs more rapidly than in individual psychotherapy. In much the same way that holistic medicine treats the entire person, not simply physical symptoms, the family-systems approach recognizes the need for family therapy when any family member is suffering. If this is a situation that applies to your family, family counseling is strongly recommended. The family-systems approach is practiced predominantly by social workers.

Good parenting requires both *time* and *consistency* in order to impart the values that you would like to instill in your children. Putting in time as a parent includes being with them on a regular basis and making an effort to get to know them better. What are their talents? What do they enjoy doing? What are they thinking about and how do they feel? Learning the answers to such questions can pay big dividends for both you and your children. In fostering their growth as individuals, it is essential to give them greater power and responsibility by allowing them to make some of their own decisions. By doing so, you will also instill confidence and trust, both in themselves and in you.

Other ways to spend time as a family are to worship together each week at church or synagogue and to designate a regularly scheduled time during the weekend for a fun activity. Take turns allowing each member to choose the activity for the day. The value of such play cannot be overemphasized. Having fun together as a family strengthens the bonds of love between each family member and defuses whatever stress or other problems may have built up during the week. Even if you cannot be with your child daily (due to being away on business or divorce, for instance), spending consistent time with them on a regular basis will help them experience the world and live their lives with the security, confidence, and caring that comes from their knowing that you love them. Despite all of its inherent struggles and perils, parenting is first and foremost an incredible gift. Appreciating that gift by regularly interacting with your children is one of the most potent means for creating community and fostering both spiritual and social healing that you will ever have.

SUMMARY

Your spiritual well-being is ultimately the most important aspect of your ability to care for yourself. It is also the dimension of holistic medicine that is most often neglected in our society. *Becoming spiritually healthy is a process of diminishing fear and increasing love while developing an awareness of soul and Spirit and allowing It to guide you to a deeper connection to other human beings.* This infinite source of compassionate and forgiving transcendent power is the essence of all life on earth and is the spark of life-force energy within each of us. The most direct path to becoming spiritually healthy is learning to love yourself. As you do, you will appreciate greater meaning and purpose in your life, experience gratitude for your many blessings, and become highly attuned to and trusting of your intuition. As you move beyond the confining restraints of your ego, you will become a more loving friend, spouse or committed partner, parent, and member of your community. In short, you will achieve the goal of holistic medicine: *to become whole,* and to experience a quality of life beyond anything you've ever imagined! Or at least beyond a score of 325 on the Wellness Self-Test.

RESOURCE GUIDE

For more information about the Arthritis Survival Program or to make an appointment with Dr. Todd Nelson, please call (303) 744-7858.

The following companies provide both information and products particularly useful for people with arthritis:

- The Arthritis Foundation: (800) 283-7800 or *www.arthritis.org*
- Aids for Arthritis, Inc.: (800) 654-0707
- MOMS Home Healthcare: (800) 232-7443
- Smith & Nephew, Inc.: (800) 558-8633 or *www.smith-nephew. com*

The following organizations offer additional information about various aspects of the Arthritis Survival Program, and provide referrals to practitioners of the many therapies that contribute to this holistic approach for treating, preventing, and curing arthritis:

HOLISTIC MEDICINE

American Board of Holistic Medicine (ABHM)
(425) 741-2996
Fax: (425) 787-8040

The ABHM is the first organization to certify physicians in Holistic Medicine (December 2000 was the first certification examination) and to create the standard of care for holistic medical practice. Provides a referral list of board-certified holistic physicians.

American Holistic Medical Association (AHMA)
6728 Old McLean Village Drive
McLean, VA 22101-3906
(703) 556-9728
Fax: (703) 556-8729

www.holisticmedicine.org (A physician referral directory is available.) The nation's oldest advocacy group (founded in 1978) devoted to promoting, teaching, and researching Holistic Medicine. Provides a list of referrals nationwide of holistic physicians (M.D.'s and D.O.'s), available on the Web site.

OSTEOPATHIC MEDICINE

American Academy of Osteopathy
3500 DePauw Blvd, Suite 1080
Indianapolis, IN 46268
(317) 879-1881

Affiliate organization representing D.O.'s who provide osteopathic manipulative treatments and/or cranial osteopathy as part of their practice.

CRANIOSACRAL THERAPY

Cranial Academy
8606 Allisonville Road, Suite 130
Indianapolis, IN 46268
(317) 594-0411
Fax: (317) 594-0411 and (317) 594-9299
Provides information and a referral list of craniosacral therapists.

Upledger Institute
11211 Prosperity Farms Road
Palm Beach Gardens, FL 33410
(407) 622-4706
Fax: (407) 622-4771

Offers training, information, and referrals.

ACUPUNCTURE/TRADITIONAL CHINESE MEDICINE

American Association for Oriental Medicine
433 Front Street
Catasauqua, PA, 18032
(610) 266-1433
Fax: (610) 264-2768

Professional association for non-M.D. acupuncturists. Offers publications and referral directory of members nationwide.

American Academy of Medical Acupuncture
58200 Wilshire Blvd., Suite 500
Los Angeles, CA 90036
(213) 937-5514

Professional association of physician acupuncturists (M.D.'s and D.O.'s). Provides educational materials, post-graduate courses, and a membership directory of members nationwide.

National Commission for the Certification of Acupuncturists
1424 16th NW, Suite 601
Washington, DC 20036
(202) 232-1404

Provides information about acupuncture and offers a test used by various states to determine competency of acupuncture practitioners.

National Acupuncture Detoxification Association
3115 Broadway, Suite 51
New York, NY 10027
(212) 993-3100

Leading organization of its kind. Conducts research on, and provides training in, the use of acupuncture to treat addiction, including alcoholism.

Qigong Institute/East-West Academy of Healing Arts
450 Sutter, Suite 916
San Francisco, CA 94108
(415) 788-2227

Provides education, training, and research about *qigong* in relation to health and healing.

BEHAVIORAL MEDICINE/ MIND-BODY MEDICINE

National Institute for the Clinical Application of Behavioral Medicine
P.O. Box 523
Mansfield Center, CT 06250
(860) 456-1153
Fax: (860) 423-4512

Provides conferences and information for practitioners.

Association for Humanistic Psychology
45 Franklin Street, Suite 315
San Francisco, CA 94102
(415) 864-8850

Provides publications about humanistic psychology and a list of referrals.

Center for Mind–Body Medicine
5225 Connecticut Avenue NW, Suite 414
Washington, DC 20015
(202) 966-7338

An educational program for health and mental health professionals, and laypeople interested in exploring their own capacities for self-knowledge and self-care. Provides educational and support groups for people with chronic illness, stress management groups, and training and programs in mind/body health care.

Mind/Body Medical Institute
New Deaconess Hospital
185 Pilgrim Road
Boston, MA 02215
(617) 632-9530

Provides research, training, and conferences related to behavioral medicine, stress reduction, yoga, and meditation.

BODYWORK/MASSAGE THERAPIES

American Massage Therapy Association
820 Davis Street, Suite 100
Evanston, IL 60201
(312) 761-2682

Provides comprehensive information on most areas of bodywork and massage, including an extensive review of the latest scientific research. Also publishes *Massage Therapy Journal,* available at most health food stores and many newsstands nationwide.

Associated Bodywork and Massage Professionals
P.O. Box 489
Evergreen, CO 80439
(303) 674-8478

Provides information and referrals.

ROLFING

International Rolf Institute
302 Pearl Street
Boulder, CO 80306
(303) 449-5903

Provides information, training, and referral directory.

REFLEXOLOGY

International Institute of Reflexology
P.O. Box 12462
St. Petersburg, FL 33733
(813) 343-4811

Provides information, training, and referrals.

CHIROPRACTIC

American Chiropractic Association
1701 Clarendon Blvd.
Arlington, VA 22209
(703) 276-8800

Professional association offering education and research into chiropractic. Also offers publications.

International Chiropractors Association
1110 North Glebe Road, Suite 1000
Arlington, VA 22201
(800) 423-4690 and (703) 528-5000

Professional association offering education and research into chiropractic. Also offers publications.

DIET AND NUTRITION

American College for Advancement in Medicine (ACAM)
23121 Verdugo Drive, Suite 204
Laguna Hills, CA 92653
(800) 532-3688

ACAM provides information about the use of nutritional supplements and a referral directory of physicians worldwide who have been trained in nutritional medicine.

American College of Nutrition
722 Robert E. Lee Drive
Wilmington, NC 28480
(919) 452-1222

Information resource for nutrition research.

Center for Science in the Public Interest
1875 Connecticut Avenue NW, Suite 300
Washington, DC 20009
(202) 332-9110
Fax: (202) 265-4954

Provides a directory of organic mail order suppliers, hormone-free beef suppliers, and general information on diet and nutrition.

American Dietetic Association
216 West Jackson, Suite 800
Chicago, IL 60606
(312) 899-0040

Provides information and certification.

International Association of Professional Natural Hygienists
Regency Health Resort and Spa
2000 South Ocean Drive
Hallandale, FL 33009
(305) 454-2220

Professional organization of physicians who specialize in therapeutic fasting.

Great Smokies Diagnostic Laboratory
63 Zillicoa St.
Asheville, NC 28801-1074
(800) 522-4762

Offers fully certified advanced assessments using over 100 diagnostic tests of digestive, immune, endocrine, nutritional, and metabolic function; supported by a comprehensive network of educational and scientific resources.

ENERGY MEDICINE

International Society for the Study of Subtle Energies and Energy Medicine (ISSSEEM)
356 Goldco Circle
Golden, CO 80401
(303) 278-2228
Fax: (303) 279-3539

Research organization; provides education and information as well as publications.

THERAPEUTIC TOUCH

Nurse Healers Professional Associates, Inc.
1211 Locust Street
Philadelphia, PA 19107
(215) 545-8079

Provides information on training, conferences, and referrals of TT practitioners. Also publishes a newsletter.

HEALING TOUCH

Colorado Center for Healing Touch, Inc.
198 Union Blvd., Suite 204
Lakewood, CO 80228
Provides information and referrals.

REIKI

Reiki Alliance
P.O. Box 41
Cataldo, ID 83810
(208) 682-3535

Provides information and referrals.

ENERGY DEVICES

Tools For Exploration
9755 Independence Avenue
Chatsworth, CA 91311
(888) 748-6657

Provides nonmedical energy machines and other devices. Free catalog available on request.

ENVIRONMENTAL MEDICINE

American Academy of Environmental Medicine
7701 E. Kellogg, Suite 625
Wichita, KS 67207
(316) 684-5500

Provides referral list of physicians practicing environmental medicine, as well as a newsletter and other information.

Human Ecology Action League (HEAL)
P.O. Box 49126
Atlanta, GA 30359
(404) 248-1898

Provide referrals to support groups that assist people suffering from environmental illness.

Immuno Labs
1620 West Oakland Park Blvd., Suite 300
Fort Lauderdale, FL 33311
(800) 321-9197

A lab specializing in allergy testing. Also provides referrals to environmental physicians worldwide.

HERBAL MEDICINE

American Botanical Council
P.O. Box 201660
Austin, TX 78720
(512) 331-8868

A nonprofit research organization and education council that serves as a clearinghouse of information for professionals and laypeople alike.

Herb Research Foundation
1007 Pearl Street
Boulder, CO 80302
(303) 449-2265

Provides research information and referrals to resources on botanical medicine worldwide. Also publishes *HerbalGram*.

HOMEOPATHY

International Foundation for Homeopathy
2366 Eastlake Avenue East, Suite 301
Seattle, WA 98102
(206) 324-8230

Provides training in homeopathy and offers referrals.

National Center for Homeopathy
801 North Fairfax, Suite 306
Alexandria, VA 22314
(703) 548-7790

Offers training in homeopathy and provides referrals.

NATUROPATHIC MEDICINE

American Association of Naturopathic Physicians
2366 Eastlake Avenue East, Suite 322
Seattle, WA 98102
(206) 323-7610

Provides information, publications, and a referral directory of naturopathic physicians. Also in the forefront in licensing of naturopaths throughout the U.S.

The Institute for Naturopathic Medicine
66½ North State Street
Concord, NH 03301
(603) 255-8844

Medical Astrology
Jonathan Keyes
(503) 231-9146
email: jonkeyes@qwest.net

A nonprofit organization promoting research about naturopathy. Offers information to professionals and laypeople as well as the general media.

PRODUCT INDEX

THRIVING HEALTH PRODUCTS

Glucosamine Plus—glucosamine sulfate and chondroitin sulfate

Collagen Support—collagen

Super Potency Essential Fatty Acids—omega-3 oils, EPA, and DHA

Calcium Supreme—high quality calcium containing glucosamine

Herbal Joint Relief—boswellia, curcumin, and ginger

Arthro Support—niacinamide and NAC

All are available through Thriving Health, Inc., at (888) 434-0033.

INDEX

Index

Index

Hahnemann, Samuel, 68
Harvard Mastery of Stress Study, 192
Hawthorn berry, 55
Hay, Louise L., 132
Healing touch resources, 203
Health, 15–16
  optimal, 16–18
  Wellness Self-Test, 19–22
Healthy Pleasures (Ornstein and Sobel), 145
Heller, Joseph, 73
Hellerwork, 73–74
Herbs, 44, 102–104
  Arthritis Survival Program, 54–56
  Chinese, 66–67
  Quick Fix, 4–5
  resources, 204–205
Hippocrates, 25, 64
Hip replacement, 13
Holistic medicine, 24–27. *See also* Arthritis Survival Program
  resources, 196
Holmes, Ernest, 128
Homeopathic medicine, 68–70
  resources, 205
Hormones, 56
House, James, 185
Huggins, Hal, Dr., 116
Humor, 144–147
Hydrogenated fats, 89
Hydrotherapy, 56
Hypoallergenic diet, 32–44

Inflammation, 9
Insulin, 86
Intimacy, 187
Intuition, 174–175
Isometric exercise, 57

Isotonic exercise, 57

Joint stress reduction, 12
Jonas, Wayne, Dr., 51
Journaling, 158–160
The Journal of the American Medical Association, 46, 159
Juice fasting, 45
Julius, Mara, Dr., 148–149

Kidney system, 67
Klass, Jared, 169
Klebsiella pneumoniae, 53
Knee replacement, 13–14
Kübler-Ross, Elisabeth, 167

LaBarge, Stephen, Dr., 157
Lactobacillus acidophilus, 53
Laughter, 146
L-glutamine, 53
Licorice root, 55
Life-force, 178
Live Better Longer, 176–177
Love, Medicine, and Miracles (Siegel), 129
Lunch
  menu suggestions, 38
  recipes, 42–44

Magnesium glycinate, 53, 102
Manganese, 53, 102
Marriage, 187–190
Massage therapy resources, 199–200
Matthews, Dale A., Dr., 168
Meadowsweet, 55
Meditation, 153–154, 170–171
Mental health, 17–18, 20–21
  optimal, 121–147
Methionine, 53

Index

ABOUT THE AUTHORS

Robert S. Ivker, D.O.

Dr. Robert Ivker is a holistic family physician and healer. He began practicing family medicine in Denver in 1972, after graduating from the Philadelphia College of Osteopathic Medicine. He completed a family practice residency at Mercy Medical Center in Denver and was certified by the American Board of Family Practice (ABFP) from 1975 to 1988. For the past fourteen years his holistic medical practice has focused on the treatment of chronic disease and the creation of optimal health. He is an Assistant Clinical Professor in the Department of Family Medicine and a Clinical Instructor in the Department of Otolaryngology at the University of Colorado School of Medicine. Dr. Ivker is a co-founder of the American Board of Holistic Medicine (ABHM) and co-creator of the first board-certification examination in holistic medicine in December 2000. He was the President of the American Holistic Medical Association (AHMA) from 1996 to 1999. Along with the four editions of the bestselling *Sinus Survival: The Holistic Medical Treatment for Sinusitis, Allergies, and Colds,* Dr. Ivker is the co-author of *The Self-Care Guide to Holistic Medicine: Creating Optimal Health* and *Thriving: The Holistic Guide to Optimal Health for Men. Arthritis Survival* is part of a Survival Guide series that also includes *Asthma Survival, Backache Survival,* and *Headache Survival,* all published by Tarcher/Putnam in 2001 and 2002. He has been married for thirty-three years to Harriet, a psychiatric social worker. They have two daughters, Julie and Carin, and live in Littleton, Colorado.

Todd H. Nelson, N.D., D.Sc.

Dr. Nelson is a naturopathic doctor and director of the Tree of Life Wellness Center in Denver, Colorado. His specialty is clinical nutrition and functional medicine. He has been serving the Denver/Boulder community for eighteen years, integrating comprehensive holistic health care through balanced, educational approaches to self-care. Dr. Nelson lectures extensively on a broad range of holistic health topics, both locally and nationally. He also teaches a corporate wellness program, Stress Mastery, to major corporations. He is the co-host of a popular radio show, HealthTime on KHOW, Colorado's number-one weekly talk show on alternative health care. Todd lives in Denver with his wife, Dixie, and four daughters.